THE REBEL MAMA'S HANDBOOK FOR (COOL) MOMS

Vol 1: Early Motherhood

ALEKSANDRA JASSEM
NIKITA STANLEY

FriesenPress

Suite 300 - 990 Fort St
Victoria, BC, V8V 3K2
Canada

www.friesenpress.com

First Edition — 2018

Writing on page 40-43 by Erica Moore

Writing on page xi-xiii and 152-155 by Meg Broadbent

Edited by Meg Broadbent

ISBN
978-1-5255-2496-7 (Paperback)
978-1-5255-2497-4 (eBook)

1. FAMILY & RELATIONSHIPS

Distributed to the trade by The Ingram Book Company

For rebellious mothers who ought to be revered,
not feared.

CONTENTS

Part 4

ON TODDLERS

Part 5

ON SIBLINGS

Part 6

ON ESCAPING

Part 7

MAMA DRAMA

THE REBEL MAMA'S
HANDBOOK FOR (COOL) MOMS

Vol 1: Early Motherhood

A Modern Conversation About
Pregnancy and Early Motherhood

FOREWORD

Meg Broadbent

I was first introduced to Aleksandra Jassem and Nikita Stanley, better known as The Rebel Mamas, when my son was 10-weeks old. I was deep in the throes of sleep deprivation at the time, and I spent my days alternating between hysterically crying, hysterically laughing, yelling at my husband, and laying dramatically on the bathroom floor.

As a first-time mom, I felt completely overwhelmed and totally alone. I had no idea what the fuck I was doing, and I was constantly on the verge of an anxiety-driven meltdown.

Why was my son crying so much? Why was he sleeping all day but never at night? Was he supposed to barf after every feed? Why was I so sad and angry all the time? Why was I bleeding like I was on the brink of death? What in the HELL was happening with my vagina?!

I needed answers, and I needed them now. I needed someone in my corner to reassure me that everything was going to be okay, to tell me that I was doing a fine job, and to hand me a properly made, slightly dirty martini.

Enter The Rebel Mamas.

When I discovered their online society of judgment-free, no-bullshit, tell-it-like-it-is moms, I suddenly felt less alone. These women understood that mothers needed a safe space to ask for help without being lectured or looked down upon. They needed to be part of a community where no one was pretending to have everything figured out, and where perfection was viewed as an amusing inside joke, not an achievable standard.

With the encouragement and support of my new mom-crew, I found the strength to pull up my adult diapers, toss my breast pump aside, put on a pair of non-maternity jeans, and start living again.

I stopped caring about getting everything right. Instead, I focused on getting through the day.

Before long, I once again recognized the person staring back at me in the mirror. Sure, I looked a little more haggard, and the circles under my eyes were darker than my coffee, but I believed in myself again. I finally realized that growing a human inside of my body, pushing it out, and managing to not accidentally kill it every day made me a hero - more than a hero! It made me a Rebel Mama.

If you picked up this book, chances are you're a Rebel Mama, too.

A Rebel Mama is a smart, brave, unapologetic bad-ass who doesn't let anyone tell her what to do or how to feel. She doesn't care what other people think; she trusts her gut and her heart. She's a confident, open-minded boss, who practices compassion and never judges another woman. Especially not another mother.

As a bonafide Rebel Mama, this book is your bible. It's your early motherhood survival guide, full of important and disgusting information that your mothers and girlfriends should have told you, but didn't. It's got advice on everything from packing a hospital bag to losing your postnatal virginity. It has tips on sleep training (have good wine on hand) and introducing solids (don't wear white). It'll teach you how to survive your first post-baby hangover and a six-hour flight with a screaming toddler. It will tell you how to look put-together, how to deal with your ever-changing breasts, and how to get five goddamn minutes to yourself.

More than anything, this book is a love letter to moms. It's not all about the kids: you still matter. Your life doesn't have to change completely the moment you get knocked up. You're a unique woman, with ideas and plans and goals, and you don't have to abandon any of them just because you've got a permanent plus one.

Motherhood is life's greatest balancing act. Raising tiny humans while holding onto your own identity and finding time for yourself is hard work, and there's no secret formula for pulling it off. No one knows what they're doing. All you can do is get up every morning and do your best. The good news? We're all in this together.

Hold onto your uteri, ladies: it's gonna be one hell of a ride.

COMMON-SENSE DISCLAIMER

Since we're about to unload a shit-ton of advice about things related to pregnancy, childbirth, nutrition, and sleep habits, among other things, we've been advised by our lawyer to include *un petit disclaimer*, so here it is:

We're not doctors. The advice in this book is based upon experience (and common sense) only.

If you have questions or concerns about your well-being or your child's health, we strongly suggest you take it up with a medically trained professional.

That is all.

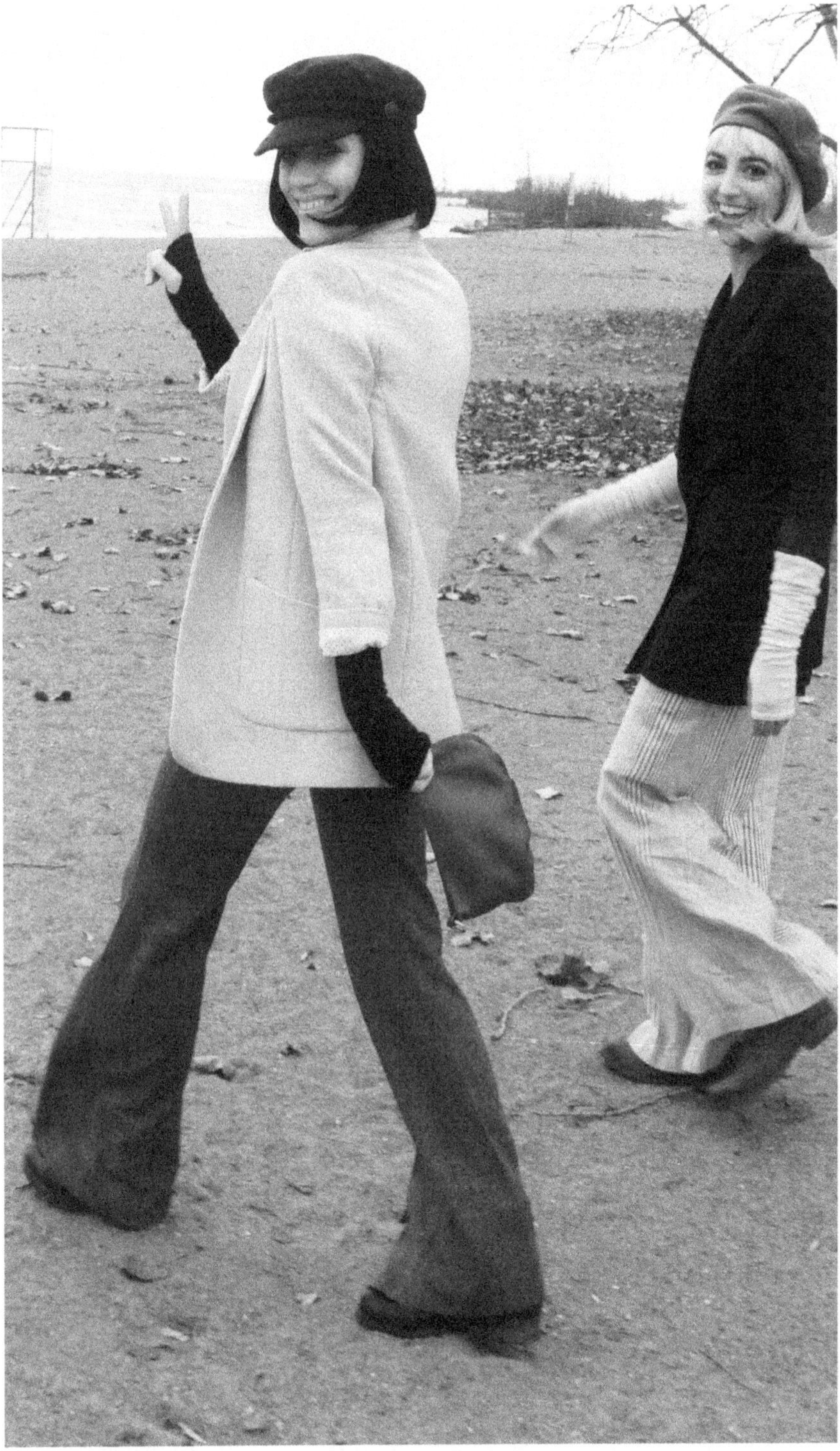

GLOSSARY OF REBEL MAMA TERMS

Occasionally, we like to employ words / acronyms that don't technically exist in the English Language. While some of their meanings are obvious, others may have you pausing to consult Google - and we certainly don't want that happening - so we've created a little glossary for you to familiarize yourself with before we begin.

In the order in which they appear in the book:

Hella: Extremely (Our second favourite unit of measurement)

AF: An abbreviation for As Fuck
(Our favourite unit of measurement)

GD: An abbreviation for Goddamn (An adjective)

FOMO: An abbreviation for Fear of Missing Out (Mostly as it relates to matters of the social variety)

INTRODUCTION:
SORRY FOR WHAT I SAID WHEN I WAS A CHILDLESS ASSHOLE

One thing we can absolutely guarantee is that once your bundle of joy arrives, you will be flooded with emotions. There will be tears, laughter, shock, and joy - sometimes all within a two-minute span. There will also be waves of embarrassment and regret, mostly pertaining to your pre-parenthood life. Among other things, you will look back on those days as the time when you said some pretty messed-up shit to (or about) your friends with kids, and you will suddenly have an overwhelming desire to dig a hole of shame and throw yourself into it forevermore.

"Did those things even come out of my mouth?
Was I an insensitive dick?"

Yes, they did, and yes, you were. Don't be too hard on yourself, though. We've all been that inconsiderate asshole at some point. But now the tables have turned, leaving you on the receiving end of a never-ending stream of commentary from your childless compadres.

Here are some eye-roll-inducing things you may hear from them in the coming months:

"I'm exhausted. I really feel it when I get less than eight hours of sleep."

"Let's go for dinner! I made a reservation for 9:30 p.m."

"Sorry we kept the baby up late! At least he'll sleep in tomorrow!"

"When I have a baby, I'm not going to let his schedule control my life. He's going to be on MY schedule."

"Hey, girl! I know I said I could be there to visit the baby at 3:00 p.m., but it's looking like it'll be closer to 5:30 p.m. Cool?"

"OMG! Learn to control your kid already!" (about a 2-year-old)

"Look at these kids with their iPads. My kids won't touch electronics until they're at least 12. Do you know how bad it is for their brains?"

"All newborns do is sleep! How can it possibly be THAT tiring?"

"I'm never having kids."

LOL / Shut-the-fuck-up, right? When you have the urge to slap these people repeatedly, take a deep breath and remember that you probably said this shit to some poor new mother back in the day as well. We too were once clueless twenty-somethings. But now we're the ladies sitting beside you at the new hipster spot in town (albeit with a 6:30 p.m. reso), yawning as we eat our dinner, and our words.

*inserts foot in mouth

Part 1
ON PREGNANCY

"Tired is the new black" – Amy Poehler

UNSOLICITED
RAPID-FIRE ADVICE

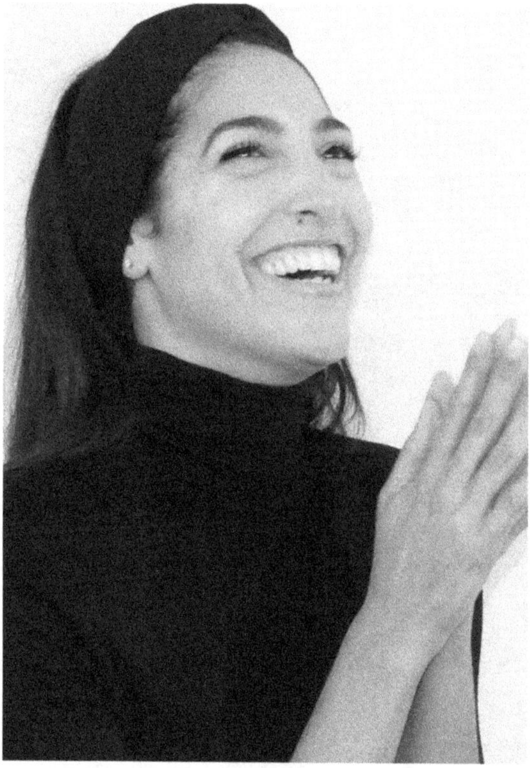

◊ You automatically win every argument just by reminding your opponent that you're currently growing another human inside your body.

◊ Making a "birth plan" is fine, but don't get too wrapped up in it. The real plan should be this: Get the baby out safely. Anything beyond that is a bonus.

- ◊ You will be bombarded with advice. People mean well, but that doesn't mean they know shit about what's right for you. Learn the subtle art of smiling and nodding.
- ◊ If you're given the okay to exercise by your doc, do it. Your body needs to be strong to get through pregnancy, labour, and delivery. Now is not the time to become a couch potato. Your postpartum self will thank you.
- ◊ At the same time, don't get too fixated on weight gain. You can get rid of the extra pounds later, if you need to. Take a deep breath and let your body do its thing; it knows what's up.
- ◊ You don't need "maternity clothes." Just go a size (or two) up. And remember, black is your best friend.
- ◊ Google "keep pants button shut with hair elastic" to make your non-maternity jeans last you through to the second trimester.
- ◊ Book. A. Trip. Pregnancy is one of the best (and last, for a while) times to get away and do fuck all in total peace.
- ◊ Tell your partner how you feel as often as possible. As much as you wish they could, they really can't read your mind. Chances are, they probably feel as scared and lost as you do.

WHEN PREGNANCY MEETS VANITY

Finding out you're pregnant is a different experience for everybody. Some women peek down at the plus sign on their pee stick and promptly log into Pinterest for inspo on how to adorably share the news with friends and family. Others (ahem, us) experience a wave of anxiety that makes them thankful they're standing beside the toilet, because they either need a place to sit down, or a place to puke.

Notwithstanding your initial reaction, once the news of an impending baby bump starts to settle in, the vain bitch inside of you will inevitably start to ask some hard-pressing questions:

"How much weight will I gain during pregnancy?"

"Will my ankles swell?"

"DOES EVERYBODY GET STRETCH MARKS?"

We'll be the first to admit that our hearts always skipped a beat at our monthly weigh-ins. Seeing the number on the scale increase by 1-2 pounds a week is kinda freaky, even for the most self-assured mamas among us. We constantly stared at our skin in the mirror at the end of the day to make sure no hormone-induced blemishes had popped up, and we religiously creeped Instagram to see how our belly sizes compared to our fellow preggos.

Like every other pregnant woman in existence, we're guessing you've been dying for someone to give you the real lowdown re: the effects of pregnancy on your bod. So, without further ado, here are some facts to calm your inner-narcissist:

CONS	PROS
Your alcohol consumption will drastically decrease.	Clean liver = glowing skin.
You're going to put on about thirty pounds during pregnancy.	You might lose about forty pounds postpartum.
For the first few months, you won't even look pregnant; you'll just look like you've overdone it on the Mexican food.	Nobody notices weight gain of anything under fifteen pounds.
You'll feel like you look fat.	You never look as fat as you feel. Seriously.
You won't be able to stay up past 10:00 p.m.	You will never miss out on your beauty rest.
Hormones will make a lot of your hair fall out postpartum.	Hormones will make your hair thick, long, and shiny AF during pregnancy.
Postpartum hair loss is often concentrated around the hairline.	A sparse hairline can be easily disguised with a heavy fringe (BONUS: Getting a new 'do' might make you feel like a superstar again!).
You will become super sensitive to smells.	You will have an automatic excuse to not take the garbage out.
Your feet might grow a little.	UM, HELLO! NEW SHOES!
Your breasts will become sensitive as they start producing milk.	You will get a sneak-peek at how you'd look with implants.
Every pregnancy is different. You may never experience any of the Pros.	Every pregnancy is different. You may never experience any of the Cons.

The most important advice we can give you is this: Don't waste your precious time worrying about how your body will change during pregnancy. It will eventually return to its original stature (or something close to it). The female form is majestic.

Having said that, on the days when you feel like total shit, a bold lipstick (Tom Ford anything) and a great hat will go a long way.

HOW TO PRODUCE A (BADASS) MATERNITY SHOOT

We have a mutual aversion to maternity shoots. The belly-cupping, the cheesy backdrops, and the unflattering lighting are enough to make any Rebel Mama cringe. When we were pregnant, all we wanted was a better, cooler way to document the amazing transformation our bodies were going through, and we're guessing that's something that you've been dreaming of as well.

That's why, with the help of photographer Ariane Laezza (the genius who executed both of our maternity portraits), we compiled a list of tips on how to turn that dream into a reality.

Work with a professional.

Friends may take beautiful photographs, but it's worth the time and money to work with an expert who has an eye for portraits (and understands the subtle art of photoshop).

Do your research.

Figure out the style of portrait you want in advance (hello, Pinterest), research photographers in your city who shoot in the same style, then ask your network for any recommendations.

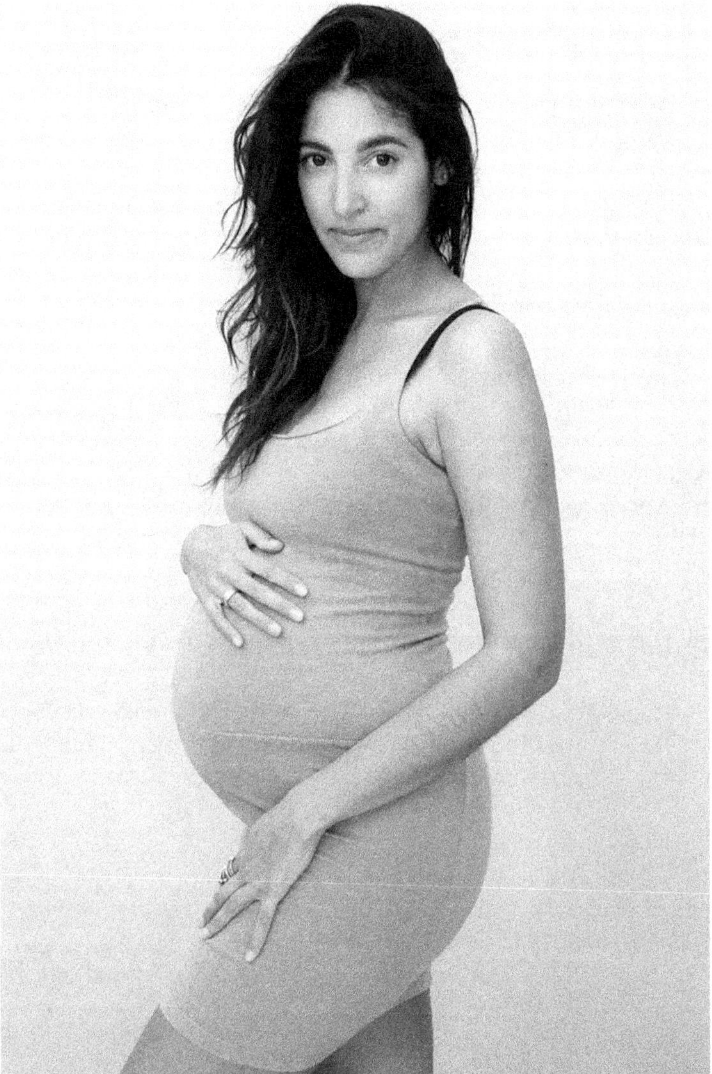

Meet with the photographer.

It's important to test out your chemistry ahead of time. The best portraits happen when you feel comfortable in the moment, so make sure you like who you're working with.

(Try to) get a good night's rest and eat well the morning of the shoot.

We know that this is easier said than done for a pregnant lady, but you want to be comfortable, rested, and energized to look your best.

Keep your wardrobe simple.

Avoid patterns, logos, and stripes. Stick to neutral colours like black, white, beige, and navy, and organic fabrics like cotton and silk. Avoid wearing over-the-top jewellery or accessories, and keep your hair and makeup natural. The goal is for you to stand out, not what you're wearing. Choose pieces that show off your growing belly-tight in some spots, flowing in others (think body con dress + loose kimono, or lace bralette + boyfriend jeans).

Ask the photographer to see a few photos during the shoot.

Once you have an idea of lighting and body positioning, turn the trust back to the photographer and allow yourself to have fun in the moment. They will guide you the rest of the way.

Get what you want.

Your photographer will likely send you some low-resolution proofs to choose from. If there are any areas of concern, bring them up. Some women have stretch marks or scars they want covered up, and it's more than ok to ask for that (it's also more than ok to embrace that shit).

Timing is everything.

If you know your home gets fantastic light in the morning, book your shoot for first thing in the a.m.

Clean your entire house.

It's a good idea to have all rooms photo-ready in case your photographer spots a corner she wants to shoot in that you'd never considered to be anything special.

Get rid of distractions.

If you have other small children at home, make sure you book your photo session with their schedule in mind, or arrange for them to go to grandma's for a few hours.

Happy shooting!

REGISTRY S.O.S.

Anyone who has stepped foot in a baby store is familiar with the copious amounts of stuff that line the shelves indefinitely. It's a multi-billion-dollar industry, and you better believe the $25 organic teething ring you're about to buy is part of it. Because we have your back, and we like keeping cash in your pocket, we've compiled a handy list of things you don't need, and a short list of things you probably want to grab.

Spend wisely, friends.

SHIT YOU DON'T NEED	SHIT YOU DO NEED
Thirty cotton swaddle blankets.	Three cotton swaddle blankets.
Two different kinds of snot suckers.	One snot sucker. Doesn't matter which one. You're sucking out boogers either way.
Super-cute diapers with an anchor pattern that you can only order online.	Diapers on sale, all of them.
Beautifully packaged, organic-lavender butt cream.	Coconut oil. Dry well and moisturize for a rash-free life.
A baby monitor that also oversees heart rate and breathing patterns.	A portable monitor with a decent camera. You will hear your baby.
A one of a kind, security blanket.	Five easily replaceable blankies that are always in stock on Amazon.
Maternity clothes. (Exception: corporate mamas)	Oversized tops and a bump band you can wear with your favourite (unzipped) jeans.
Pink hair clips and headbands as proof that your child is a girl.	The courage not to give a shit.
The top five "best-selling" baby books.	Your mom, your mom friends, your gut, and this book.
A stack of remarkably-overpriced onesies with witty slogans.	Ten neutral onesies. People will gift you with the novelty items.

SHIT YOU DON'T NEED	SHIT YOU DO NEED
The wrong breastfeeding pillow.	The right breastfeeding pillow (if you even need one at all), purchased after meeting your baby and learning what kind of support he or she needs.
A pricey brand-name diaper bag with all the bells and whistles.	A simple black nylon bag with a few compartments. (BONUS: It will double as a gym or travel bag later on.)
Infant shoes.	Infant socks.
A $400 Scandinavian high chair.	A $25 IKEA high chair.
A $120 colourful, ABC play mat from the boutique baby shop.	A $30 black and white gym mat from the internet.
A hand-me-down playpen that feels a bit flimsy.	A bomb-ass 4MOMS playpen that you will use for sleepovers and travel for years. Worth every penny.
A picturesque Restoration Hardware bassinet.	The bassinet that comes with your 4MOMS playpen.
A designer car seat that's worth the same as an actual car payment.	Any $150 car seat. They're all safe. Get one that fits in your car.
Nursing clothes.	Can you pull your tit out of it? It's a nursing top.
A hip baby wardrobe that costs a fortune and won't fit in two months.	Hand-me-downs that make your soul (and the earth) happy. It's never too early to cultivate a love of vintage.
A Jolly Jumper.	The desire to exercise your arms.
A thousand toys and stuffed animals.	Open access to the Tupperware drawer. Throw in some wooden spoons as an added bonus.
A baby-wipe warmer.	Seriously?
A Diaper Genie.	A small pail and garbage bags. Take them out every day for a routine that's far less disgusting.
A UFO chair that plays music and vibrates.	A BABYBJÖRN bouncer. The aesthetic won't mess with your décor, and it's silent.
A $1000 walnut crib from the UK (we're both guilty).	An IKEA crib that does exactly the same job.

THE MYTHICAL HORNY PREGNANT LADY

Anyone who's ever watched a movie or a TV show that involves a pregnant character is probably familiar with the concept of The Horny Pregnant Lady. She's large and in charge, and she just can't get enough of that D!

Right.

Outside of Hollywood's hilariously inaccurate portrayal of pregnant women, may we ask where in the hell these libidinous women are hiding?

We're sure there are a few women out there who still wanna get down after getting knocked up. If you're able to feel like a mega babe while another human being does somersaults in your gut, we tip our hats to you, you sly dog. In our experience, however, most pregnant women are usually thinking some combination of the following: Don't touch me, I feel fat, and I will cut you.

The literature out there supporting the existence of The Horny Pregnant Lady is endless. If you type "pregnancy and libido" into Google, a shit-ton of articles will pop up claiming that pregnancy kicks a gal's sex drive into attack mode. If you read through online forum posts about the same topic, however, the discussions consistently centre around LOWERED libidos [insert deep-in-thought emoji here].

This is a problem, folks.

All this misleading talk about The Horny Pregnant Lady is making the non-horny pregnant ladies feel like sex-hating weirdos. What's worse, a lot of these mamas-to-be feel guilty, and they worry that their temporary lack of desire will send their partners running into the arms (or vagina) of a more "eager" (read: not bloated and nauseous) lover.

That's bullshit.

First of all, if you trust your partner enough to make a baby with you, you should damn well trust them enough to stick around and hold your hand while you grow that baby in your uterus for the better part of a year. Second of all, women do NOT need yet ANOTHER thing to make us feel guilty / worried / shitty / whatever.

Instead, let's band together in our collective unhorniness. Let's make a deal to be frank and honest about our personal experiences when it comes to (not having) sex during pregnancy (and postpartum, which is a whole other story - see page 40).

If you're reading this right now thinking, THIS IS ME! I'M THE LEAST HORNY PREGNANT LADY EVER!, you are most definitely not alone. The way pregnancy is portrayed on film and TV is garbage (How "funny" is it watching labour scenes when you've experienced REAL labour?), so don't let any of those fake, airbrushed, sex-hungry bitches make you feel bad about yourself, your sex life, or your relationship. Go grab a doughnut and spoon with your body pillow. Your libido will return in due time.

BABYMOON IT UP

Assuming your pregnancy isn't high-risk, and your doctor or midwife has given you the green light to travel, we urge you to get out there and do it (especially if you're pregnant with your first child).

You won't have much (if any) precious alone time once the baby arrives, so we beg you to take advantage. You may be thinking to yourself that you'll just travel later avec bébé. You can (and should) do that as well, but we promise you it'll be a bazillion times less restful for everyone involved. You can also take solo trips down the road, of course, but they will be shorter and will require a lot more planning.

In case you need that extra nudge before clicking "BOOK NOW," we've compiled a list of reasons for you to get out there and nap in another country.

- Salt water is God's gift to pregnant women. Because you can float, all the extra baggage you've been hauling around will suddenly drift away and render you weightless.

- Fretting about your current non-bikini body is a non-issue. A glowing pregnant belly silhouetted against a sunset or ocean backdrop is straight-up Goddess material.

- Travel destinations make are ideal locations for spontaneous maternity photoshoots. In case you forgot what Paris looks like.

- You will sleep more peacefully being away from your to-do list and your mother's round-the-clock calls and emails.

- You will reconnect with your partner (especially if you can muster the willpower to disconnect from your phone).

- If Europe is your vibe, adhering to the local culture and customs will work quite well in your favour. The Italians and the French will shoo away your alcohol and pasteurization concerns, and have you sipping the finest wines and eating the richest cheeses in no time.

- You have a wonderful excuse to shop, since everything can be considered a token and souvenir of this incredible moment in your life. Especially that red YSL clutch.

Calm and relaxed mama = calm and relaxed baby. So go on - get out of here, and get your chill on. You deserve it.

THAT HOSPITAL BAG AIN'T GONNA PACK ITSELF

Ah, packing the old hospital bag. A sure sign that you've almost reached the light at the end of the long pregnancy tunnel.

Congratulations! It's nearly go-time.

As ladies who have a penchant for both comfort and practicality, when we packed our own hospital bags for the first time, under the tutelage of a shitty (but very popular) baby-prep book, we were left wishing that we'd just asked some of our savvy girlfriends what they had packed instead. Now we're in the position of being those savvy girlfriends for you, so we wrote that shit down, and we're passing it on.

For Mama

- ID, hospital card, insurance information, debit/credit card, signed documents you've been instructed by your doctor or midwife to bring

- 2 adult diapers (in case you experience avalanche-like lochia bleeding) #glamour

- 4 pairs of maternity underwear (the high-waisted, granny-panty ones that won't bother your incision site or your episiotomy stitches)

- 10 monster pads (yes, this goes for C-section mamas as well)

- 4 breast pads (in case your milk decides to come in while you're there)

- 1 nursing bra (easy boob access is now your top priority)

- 1 nightgown + 1 robe (Word to the wise: Bring only things that go down to your knees. You'll want something to cover your still-there belly, as well as your adult diapers, as you roam the halls.)

- Loose sweatpants + a light zip-up hoodie (easy nursing/ skin-to-skin access)

- 1 going-home outfit (long black cardigan + black maternity tights #allblackeverything)

- 3 pairs of socks

- Flip flops (in case you decide to shower)

- Sleep mask (in case you want to attempt a nap during the day)

- Toiletries:

  Toothbrush + toothpaste
  Face wash + moisturizer
  Deodorant
  Hair elastics + bobby pins
  Makeup (just the basics, if anything)
  Shower cap (save hair-washing for
  the comfort of your own home)
  Chapstick (hospital air is dry AF)

For your Partner

- Hopefully they can manage to pack their own socks, undies, and change of clothes

Just for Comfort

- Your own pillows—one for you, one for your partner (both in NON-WHITE LINENS, so they don't get confused with hospital crap)

- 1 blanket for your partner (who has to sleep on a shitty chair or possibly the floor)

- 2 towels—one in case you decide to shower/wash your face, and one for the car so you can sit on it during the drive to the hospital / birthing centre / middle of the woods

- Ear plugs (in case you don't land a private room)

Food + Drink

- Water (SO PARCHED)

- Coconut water or anything else that's filled with electrolytes (SO, SO PARCHED)

- Dried fruit + nuts (Need energy. Need fibre. Hate hospital food.)

- Granola bars

- Oranges, apples, bananas, pears, grapes (easy to eat / full of vitamins and fibre / don't require a fridge)

- Mints

For The Baby (!)

- CAR SEAT (DO NOT forget this one)

- 15 newborn diapers

- Wipes (for the inevitable gross black poo)

- Fold-up change pad
- Coconut oil (in lieu of diaper cream)
- 2 swaddling blankets (yes, they come wrapped in a blanket, but you'll like using your own.)
- 2 tiny cotton hats (keep that heat in! Also, newborn heads are gunky, and they look cuter when you cover them up.)
- 2 newborn onesies
- 1 warm blanket (for the car ride home)
- 2 burp cloths (in case visitors attempt to hold him while sporting a scratchy sweater or smelling like they've bathed in cologne.)
- 2 infant washcloths (we don't know why, but these things ALWAYS come in handy.)
- 1 pair of infant mittens (or just newborn socks - keep those razor-sharp claws on lock down)

Things To Keep In Mind

- When packing clothes, always ask yourself, "Can I easily whip my boob out of this?" If the answer is no, pack something else.
- Remind any visitors to come bearing food. (Don't be shy about asking for exactly what you want.)
- Also remind everyone to stop for good coffee before they walk through your recovery room door. Trust us.

Happy packing!

THE REBEL MAMA'S CODE OF CONDUCT

At this point, you may still be blissfully unaware of all the drama that plagues mommy groups, both on and offline. People seem to have a painfully hard time keeping their mouths shut when it comes to other mothers' parenting decisions. Rebel Mamas don't get caught up in that shit.

Sure, it's tempting to judge. It's natural for us to think that our way is the right way, and that every other way is inherently wrong. But at the end of the day, none of us know jack about other people's lives, so most of our thoughts and opinions should be kept to ourselves.

Rule #1: THOU SHALT NOT JUDGE ANOTHER WOMAN'S BIRTHING CHOICE

There are lots of ways to have a baby: in a hospital, in a tub in your living room, drugged up (and happy about it), drug-free (and happy about it), drug-free (and mad about it), etc. The way a child is brought into the world is nobody's business but the woman doing the heavy lifting.

Rule #2: THOU SHALT NOT JUDGE ANOTHER FAMILY'S FEEDING PRACTICES

Breastfeeding and formula feeding are both great ways to make sure babies remain alive and fed, which is all that matters. People make decisions about feeding practices based on their own unique set of circumstances. Don't say shit about it to them, ever.

Rule #3: THOU SHALT NOT JUDGE ANOTHER FAMILY'S SLEEP CHOICES

Whether you choose to co-sleep, sleep-train, or not sleep at all does not determine how good a parent you are. When it comes to sleep practices, everyone is just doing whatever works best for them to make it through the night.

Rule #4: THOU SHALT NOT JUDGE ANOTHER FAMILY BASED ON ITS COMPOSITION

Some people want one kid. Some people want eight kids. Some people want no kids. Some people want to raise their kids by themselves. Some people want to live in a commune and raise their children collectively. None of this has anything to do with you.

Rule #5: THOU SHALT NOT JUDGE ANOTHER MOTHER … EVER

If you ever find yourself in a situation where you're tempted to fall down the judgment rabbit hole, take a step back. Remind yourself that everyone's doing their best, just like you are, and redirect your energy back to something positive and useful (loving your family and making the best decisions for their overall well-being is a great place to start).

◊◊◊

And now that that's out of the way, let's continue.

Part 2
ON POSTPARTUM

"Don't tell your kids you had an easy birth or they won't respect you.
For years I used to wake up my daughter and say, 'Melissa, you ripped me to shreds.
Now go back to sleep!'"

– Joan Rivers

UNSOLICITED
RAPID-FIRE ADVICE

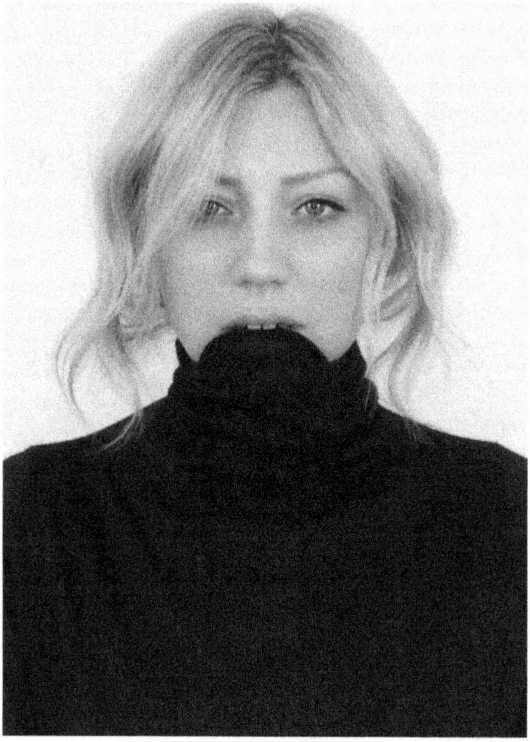

◊ Page the nurse or call the midwife incessantly during the first few days after birth. You will miss them when they're gone.

◊ Take care of yourself, and let others take care of you. Now is not the time to be a hero.

◊ Hire someone to clean your house if you can, even just for the first three months. Dust bunnies should be the least of your concerns right now.

◊ There will be a LOT of blood coming out of your vagina for a while, no matter how you gave birth. It's totally normal. So is some clotting. If you're freaked out, mention it to ANY doctor you see in the first few weeks (yes, even your kid's pediatrician, since you're there all the damn time anyway). They can help you gauge whether it's something that requires further medical attention.

◊ Don't kill your partner. It is tempting, but try to resist. They will become very useful when the baby is more active.

◊ If sex is on the agenda in the first few months postpartum (with the green light from your doc / midwife / doula, of course), come prepared with a Costco-sized container of lube. You will need it.

◊ Wet some pads and stick them in the freezer. Once fully chilled, pop one of those suckers into your giant panties for some sore-vag relief.

◊ Stay hydrated! Upping your water intake will help ease post-birth water retention, keep your milk supply up, and generally make you feel less like death.

◊ Don't feel guilty passing your baby off to other people when they come to visit. That is LITERALLY why they came over. Let them hold your child and go do something for yourself. Take a shower (wash your hair while you're in there) or go grab a proper bite to eat.

◊ If you fall victim to postpartum hair loss (solidarity, sister), a little hairspray + a regular toothbrush can help to slick down those pesky baby hairs once the regrowth starts.

◊ Have lanolin nipple cream on hand. You will cherish it forever as your most beloved boob Chapstick. (It also makes for the best actual lip Chapstick / gloss ever.)

LABOUR AND DELIVERY: IT PROBABLY WON'T GO ACCORDING TO PLAN (AND THAT'S FINE)

There was a time in our pregnancies when all we did was send birthing videos back and forth to each other.

We were both entering our third trimesters, and we were freaking out. As usual, we opted to confront our fears with facts, and went crazy doing labour and delivery research to determine the best possible way to give birth. We both decided that having a "natural" birth in a hospital was the way to go.

When D-Day arrived, we felt prepared AF. We did breathing exercises. We visualized our bodies opening like mystical portals to the unknown. We assumed that, after just a few hours, we'd be in the throes of uneventful, predictable, (dare we say) blissful vaginal births.

Oh, the naiveté!

We both ended up on operating tables due to last-minute, emergency circumstances, and our babies were both born via C-section.

Our deliveries were nothing like the ones we'd envisioned. But when all was said and done, we still ended up with cute, pink, crying babies in our arms. The hardest part was coming to terms with the fact that, no matter how hard we had tried and hoped and planned, in the end, it was all out of our control.

That's what we want you to keep in mind when you're thinking about giving birth. When it comes to your labour and delivery, not everything will go exactly according to plan, and that's okay. No matter what's in store for you, that baby is coming out, one way or another. And whatever way that may be, remember: You can to do this. Women are strong as fuck. YOU are strong as fuck! Strut into that hospital / birth centre / tub in the middle of your living room feeling fierce and empowered.

Now is not the time to worry. Now is the time to breathe, go with the flow, listen to your body, trust your intuition, and heed the advice of your chosen medical professional, who (by the way) has dedicated his/her life to learning about the very task you're about to undertake. Rest easy, Mama. You're in good hands.

You've already come so far. The finish line is in sight. Don't worry about the exact way that you'll be crossing it. Just do whatever it takes to get to the other side.

We'll be cheering for you the whole time, and waiting to celebrate with a lot of sushi and sake.

LET HER HEAL

The incredible transformation from maidenhood to motherhood is one that is generally taken too lightly. In North America specifically, there remains a deep lack of understanding about the postpartum experience. Hormones are out of whack, causing major emotional ups and downs; sleep deprivation is a monster than can wreak havoc on even the most calm and collected among us; and the feeling of isolation that a new mother experiences when the last visitor leaves and her partner heads back to work is completely overwhelming.

No woman can survive this time alone. Every new mother needs help, love, and the time and space to heal. Asking for help, however, is often the last thing on a woman's mind when she's in the throes of the fourth trimester, and even if she does consider it, it can be hard to properly vocalize her needs. That's why we wrote the following letter for all the brave women out there who have just brought new life into the world.

Pass it on.

DEAR SPOUSES, PARTNERS, FRIENDS, LOVED ONES, PARENTS, IN-LAWS, AND EVERYBODY ELSE:

When the new mom in your life arrives home with the family's new pride and joy, please, let her heal.

Only days or even hours ago, she either pushed a watermelon-sized child out of a pea-sized hole in her body, or a baby was forcefully removed from her abdomen (as her organs lay in a tray beside her). Let her heal.

She looks in the mirror and sees a woman she doesn't recognize. Her stomach is soft, her eyes are tired, her skin is pale, and her cheeks are swollen. She is afraid of her own reflection. Let her heal.

She's starving. Her body is the only source of nutrition for two humans now. She's burning hundreds of calories per day just producing milk. Make sure she has a ton of water, and healthy, whole foods available to her at all times, and let her heal.

She needs to feel fresh air on her face, but she's not strong enough to go for a walk. Lay her in bed, take the baby, bring her a cup of tea, open the bedroom windows, and let her heal.

She is prone to panic, anxiety, shock, and depression right now. She's dying to "bounce back," but it's not happening fast enough for her. Tell her she's doing great, and let her heal.

Don't dismiss her cries for help as weakness. Don't assume she's complaining, and never tell her to 'suck it up' or 'get over it'. Doing so will make her wish she had the strength to strangle you (and one day down the road, she will). Give her all the energy and patience you can muster, and let her heal.

Please, everyone: Let her heal. We promise that if you do she'll be a stronger mother and woman, and everyone stands to benefit from that. Especially her.

BOOB TALK

Pregnancy and postpartum kick a woman's boobs into overdrive, resulting in a myriad of changes over a short period of time (thanks, hormones). They start out perky and full and they end up as shells of their former selves (little pancake boobs are actually very en vogue right now, so at least there's that).

If there's one thing that pregnancy and nursing have taught us about our tatas, it's that they're legitimately, mind-bendingly magical. Remind yourself of that as you watch them transform over the coming months. And fear not, your nips will go back to their original size, eventually (sort of).

Here's what to expect:

	BEFORE PREGNANCY	DURING PREGNANCY	POSTPARTUM
YOUR AREOLAS	Pretty. Puffy. Average-sized. A few shades darker than your skin tone.	HUGE. Flat. Several shades darker than your skin tone. Sensitive.	Still HUGE. A million shades darker than your skin tone. Hella sensitive.

	BEFORE PREGNANCY	DURING PREGNANCY	POSTPARTUM
YOUR NIPPLES	Perhaps inverted. Perhaps standing at attention. Nothing to write home about.	Enlarged. Occasionally leaking some yellowish fluid (it's colostrum, which is totally normal). Often tingly.	HUGE. Sticking out like little straws. Maybe leaking milk. Maybe cracked. Maybe bleeding. Super sensitive. Usually have a baby hanging from them. *Pro tip: Cure cracked nipples by allowing some breast milk to air dry on them. If it's really bad: lanolin cream.
YOUR BOOBS	Perky. Cute. Enjoy freedom. May not require much support.	Engorged. Veiny. Tingly. Require moderate to significant support.	Bigger than they've ever been before. Occasionally lumpy. Prone to clogged ducts. (If you get one, warm compresses and massages in a hot shower are your best friends.) Incredibly veiny. So heavy you'll want a hammock rather rather than a bra to support them Painful.

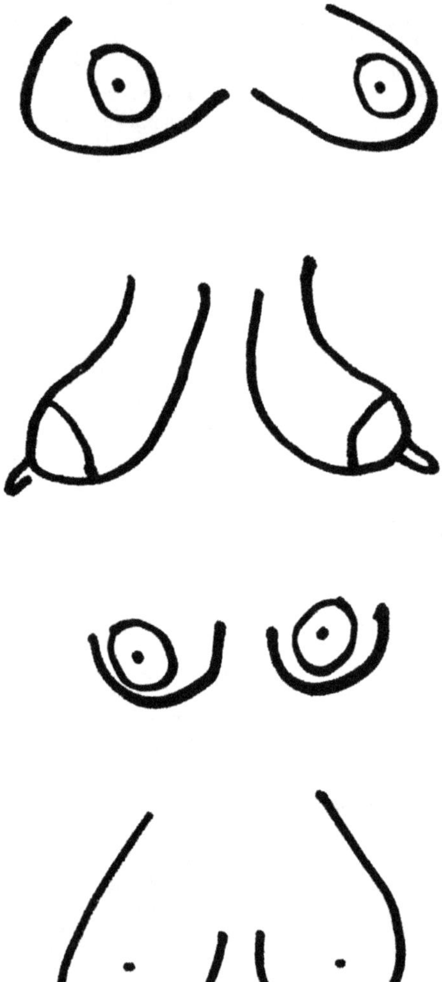

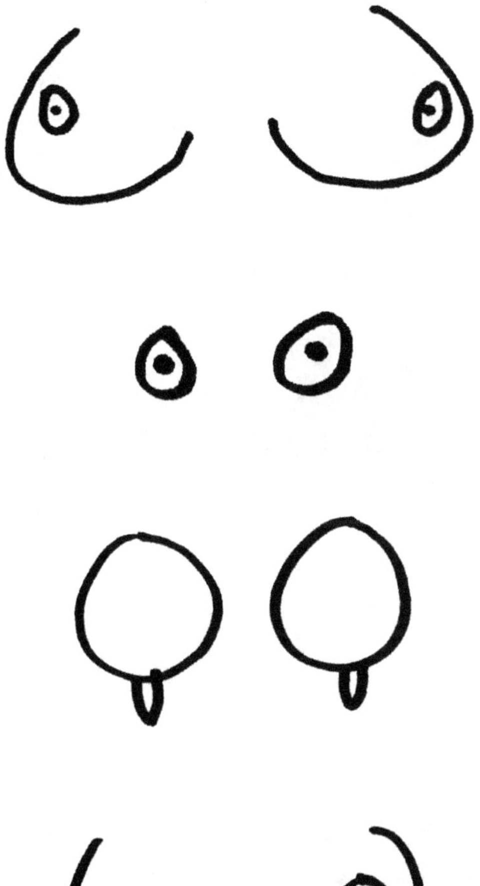

MAMA:
THE (UNINTENTIONALLY) NEW & IMPROVED YOU

We're never going to tell you that having a baby is all sunshine and rainbows. There is, however, one major perk: This mom-life that you've been living lately is slowly but surely turning you into a better human being. A more tired human being, but a better one nonetheless. Here's how:

YOU WAKE UP HELLA EARLY

For most of our lives, we hit snooze repeatedly on our alarm clocks every morning. That changed the day we got human alarm clocks that didn't come with snooze buttons and went off at the crack of dawn. At first, we hated it. Over time, however, we came to discover that morning (you know, all those hours before noon?) is a sacred time of day. It's quiet, it's calm, and the lighting is fabulous. There's no better time to reflect on yesterday and set the tone for today. Another bonus of waking up early: by 10:00 p.m., you can't keep your damn eyes open, so you actually GO TO SLEEP.

BREASTFEEDING FORCES YOU TO BE HEALTHY AF

Since we knew that whatever we put into our bodies was going to end up in our baby's milk, we suddenly became super health-conscious. We try to consume produce at every meal, we get our omegas, healthy fats, and fibre in as frequently as possible, and we're generally aware of what's going down the old hatch. We also consume less alcohol and drink a lot more water, which alone has made us look and feel healthier. There's also the added bonus of breastfeeding burning approximately 500 calories a day. Hello, skinny jeans.

YOU WALK ALL AROUND THE GD TOWN

When you have a baby, you'll walk. A lot. When we had newborns, we walked out of boredom, and because we needed to get out of the house so we wouldn't go stir crazy. As a result, we started to accidentally get at least an hour of cardio in every day just trying to kill time. The thing about cardio is that it becomes addictive after a while. To this day, we both crave the rhythm of a good walk and often jump at any opportunity to take a pavement break.

YOU FINALLY WHITTLE DOWN YOUR INNER-CIRCLE

When you have a kid, making social plans is such a bitch that it very quickly makes you realize who really matters to you. The amount of energy it takes to arrange for a babysitter, pump breast milk, organize all the baby's stuff, and get ourselves ready and out the door made us extremely picky about who we made the effort to spend time with. The only people left on your guest list will be the ones you genuinely love.

YOU CLEAN YOUR HOUSE LIKE A BOSS

Having kids has made us lean, mean, super-efficient cleaning machines. You know how you used to get home from work sometimes, with only a thirty-minute window to clean your house before your friend came over, and you were always shocked at how fast you could be when you had a firm cleaning deadline? Welcome to Mom Life. Except instead of a social engagement providing the timeline, it's the dreaded end of nap-time.

YOU'RE A MULTITASKING HERO

Multitasking: if you were good at it before, now you're a bloody expert. Not only did motherhood show us that we're able to accomplish a million things simultaneously, but it also taught us that anything we thought required the use of both hands only can actually be done with one.

YOU BECOME AN ALL-AROUND BETTER PERSON

First, there's empathy: Having babies made us understand that parenting is hard AF. We now realize that everyone is trying their best, and everyone deserves love and compassion - both other parents and other children.

We've also become less selfish: whatever it takes to make baby feel safe, secure, loved, and happy, we do it, no matter what. Finally, babies are incredibly humbling. Our kids forced us to face the fact that we often don't know what the hell we're doing, but for the first time in our lives, we know without a doubt that we're doing our best, because we're doing it for them.

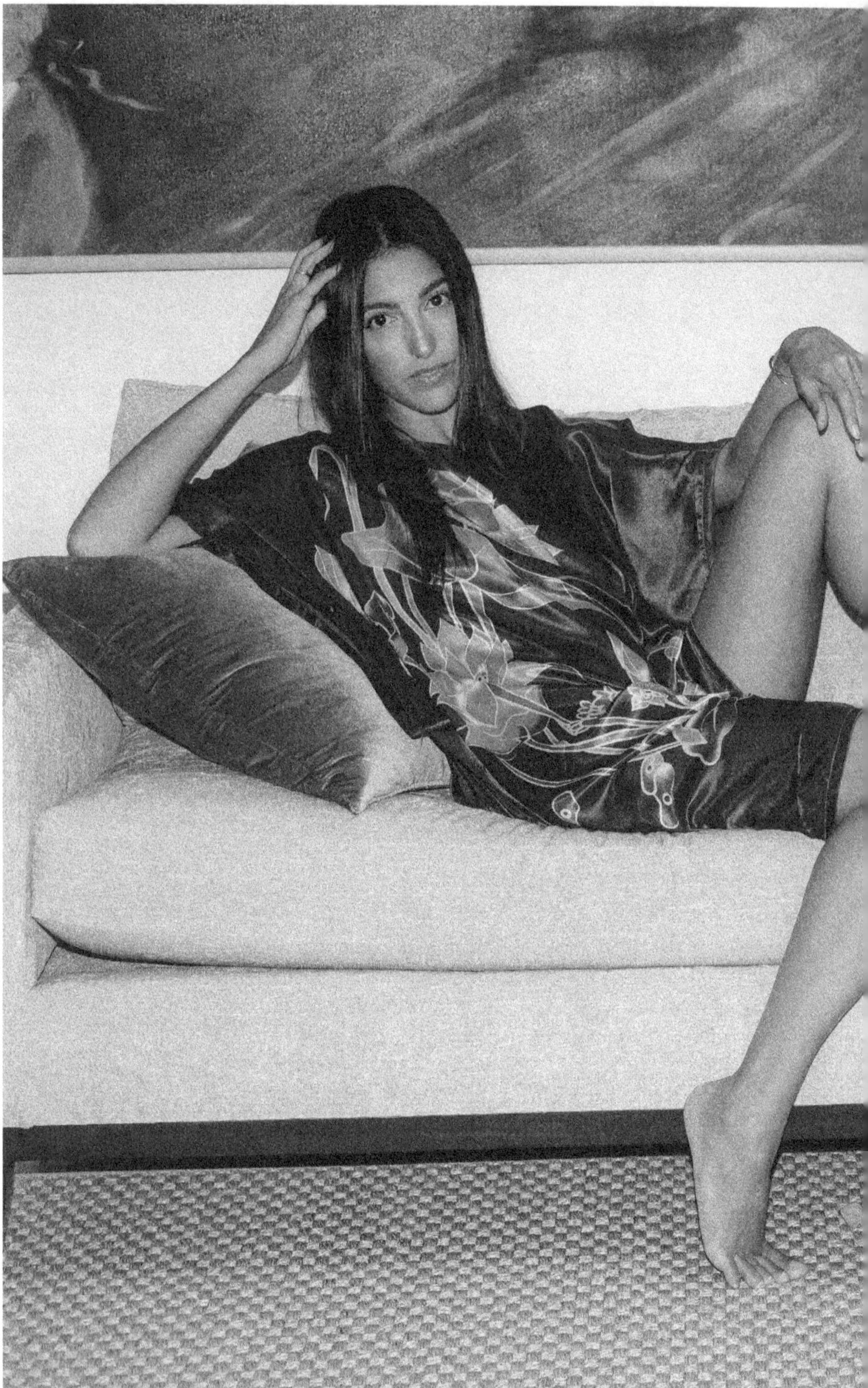

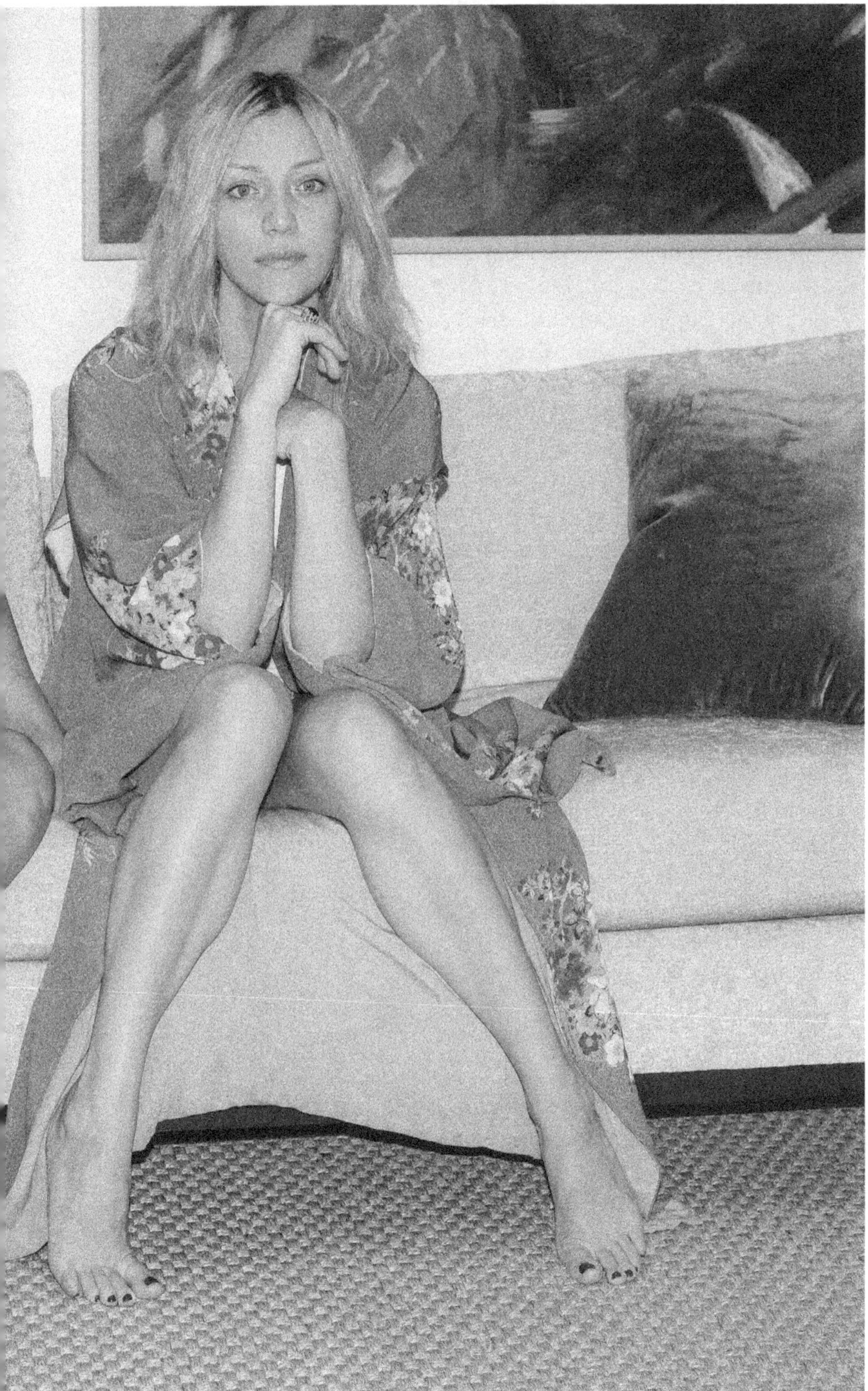

Story-time with (our friend) Erica Moore

LOSING YOUR POSTNATAL VIRGINITY

I was so convinced that my vagina would be demolished after childbirth that I spent close to $100 on a makeshift repair kit: plus-size adult diapers, perineum-shaped ice packs, and Tucks antiseptic wipes. Although labour was an insane thirty-six hours, with an epidural that ONLY froze my legs (thank you, modern science), my vagina somehow came out of it relatively unscathed.

Three-days postpartum, I went for a walk around the block. One-week postpartum, I took a longer stroll through the park. Two-weeks postpartum, I laced up my running shoes for a five-kilometre walk with the stroller. Physically, I felt great—rejuvenated and ambitious.

By week three, I felt ready to party again. My midwife said I should wait to have sex until week six to avoid infection, but on week four, baby and I took an afternoon walk to our local drugstore and found ourselves standing in the condom aisle. Feeling like a sheepish teenager perusing the possibilities of protection, I grabbed a dozen "thin silk" lubricated condoms. I purchased a chocolate bar and some cleaning products too, to make my checkout a little less awkward for everyone involved.

On the walk home, I listened to some old Usher tracks and sent my husband a text:

"Let's have sex tonight."

The evening unfolded like any other, with shitty diapers, breast pumping, and a lacklustre dinner eaten while taking turns bouncing a newborn in our laps. Around 8:00 p.m., I slipped away to prepare my bod for postnatal coitus. I shaved my armpits, legs, and toes. I considered tackling my lady bush, but realized that my razor wasn't sharp enough for that jungle.

I took a long look at myself in the mirror. I wasn't a slender gal to begin with, so I wasn't so much saddened by the extra pounds I had put on during pregnancy as I was disturbed by the way they now positioned themselves on my body. My chub, previously full and tight, now looked like flesh-coloured bread loaves stapled to my belly. My nipples had starburst over my breasts without any clearly definitive ending points.

I decided to draw attention upward to my face by putting a little makeup on. I plucked the three chin hairs that had returned since pregnancy. I even put a little foundation on my boobs to tone down the nipple extravaganza.

I found a pair of sexy underwear. As I was trying to hike them up, my hands literally ripped through the lace as if I were The Incredible Hulk. NEXT. I found another pair and managed to get fully inside of them, only to realize that they made my butt look like it was holding its breath. NEXT. I finally found a plain, black-cotton thong. It was so old that the crotch was just a few threads held together by luck and magic, but at least it fit.

I slipped into a black sheer negligee that I used to wear pre-pregnancy. My breasts were heaving to the point of discomfort, but my cleavage looked Elizabethan in a sexy way, so I decided to endure. I got into bed and waited for Husband.

I finally saw him coming up the stairs with the baby in his arms. Oh, right. The baby. The baby is now part of the sexy equation. Although I'd like to pretend that being a new mom has me feeling blessed 24/7, it simply isn't true. There are moments where I think, He's cute, but he's also a bit of a drag. This was one of those moments.

Husband looked at me and recalled our earlier text exchange, finally clueing in. He lifted an eyebrow as he gently lowered the baby into the bassinet next to our bed. "You look great, babe."

I'm not in the business of writing erotica, so I will spare you the explicit details, but let's just say we got down to business. At one point, Husband looked up at me to say something smooth, but I couldn't hear anything, because all I could see was my face / nipple foundation brushed across his cheek. I chose not to ruin the moment and simply pretended like it wasn't there.

Finally, it was time for the sex. We were doing this. I was about to lose my postnatal virginity.

Me: "Go slow."

My inner-monologue: I guess this is okay. I'm not very wet. I think breastfeeding dries you out. Is that a thing? He doesn't seem to notice. Is it weird that we're having sex right now with the baby in the same room? Can the baby see us? No, it's not weird. I'm a modern woman. This is how it's done. This is probably very European of us.

Me: "You can go a bit faster."

My inner-monologue: Okay, this feels familiar. Sex feels the same. Does it feel the same for him? Is he taking longer than normal? Oh shit, maybe I'm super stretched out and it's terrible. Maybe I'm different now, and I'll never be as good. I used to be really good. Maybe I was never THAT good though? I'll ask…

Me: "Is it good? Is it the same as it was?"

Husband: "It's great ... it feels really good."

Baby: "SQUAWK."

My inner-monologue: Oh shit, the baby made a noise. He's going to cry. If he cries, do we stop? Is it child abuse if we keep going until we finish? What if he made that noise because a blanket was somehow kicked over his face? Why isn't he making the noise again? Maybe he's dead. I bet he's dying right now, and we're here just boning. We're the kind of negligent parents you'd see in a movie like *Trainspotting.*

When the police ask what happened, do we lie? Or do we say we were having sex while our baby quietly suffocated a few feet away? They'll ask why I had sex before the recommended six weeks. Oh my god.

Baby: "Bahhhgrrggg!"

My inner-monologue: Okay, good. That sounded normal and lively. In fact, it sounded super cute, like he's babbling. He's advanced. I was really hoping he'd get my propensity for language and articulation. What a young scholar. I need to call more daycares, get him on more wait lists. Montessori, even. Who am I kidding? We can't afford that. We can't even afford to buy a house in this stupid city. I'm a terrible mother.

Husband: "I'm getting close."

My inner-monologue: Oh yeah, sex! Is that a blackhead on Husband's shoulder? How long has that been there? I wonder if he'll let me look at it after.

Husband: "Are you close as well?"

Me: "I think so?"

My inner-monologue: Nope. I'm like a good ten minutes away. Oh well, I can always take care of things on my own later…

Husband orgasms and rolls onto his back.

Baby: "Wahh, wahh, waaaahhhh!!!"

I hopped out of bed, ran to the bassinet, and was greeted by a wailing newborn baby. I scooped him up and brought him back into the bed where his parents' sinful deeds were likely still detectable by a forensic light.

Husband: "We've still got it, babe."

Me: "Yeah, we sure do."

THE FIVE STAGES OF POSTPARTUM HAIR LOSS

There are few things in life more traumatic than hopping into the shower to wash your hair, only to glance down and see that half of that amazing mane you sported during pregnancy has dislodged from your scalp and is now swirling down the drain, disappearing deep into the abyss.

If you're in the throes of this fresh hell right now, you are not alone. The hair loss you're experiencing is horrible, but luckily, it isn't permanent.

Behold: The Five Universal Stages of Postpartum Hair Loss.

STAGE ONE: DENIAL

You've recently given birth and some asshole makes an off-the-cuff remark to you along the lines of, "Has your hair started falling out yet?"

Hair? Falling … out? Pardon?

You start frantically googling "hair loss after birth," and you're thrilled to discover that apparently, some women's hair is not affected by fluctuating hormone levels. VICTORY! You convince yourself that you are one of those women. Your baby is already two-months-old, after all, and your mane remains intact. You actually believe that you've escaped the horror. You are wrong.

STAGE TWO: THE HORROR

One day, when your baby is anywhere from two to seven-months-old, you'll be taking a shower, washing your hair for the first time in a long time, and as you're rinsing out your conditioner, it will happen: Entire clumps of hair will just detach themselves from your head.

Your first thought will be "OMG, the drain!" So, you'll try to catch the clumps as they swirl about the tub, scooping them up and plastering them onto the shower wall. As you look at the disgusting abstract hair-art you've created, you'll suddenly realize that you are not the one percent. This is happening. Then you will cry. A lot.

STAGE THREE: BALD

Okay, bald may be a bit of an overstatement, but balding is pretty accurate. Goodbye, baby hairs. Goodbye, normal hairs that lived adjacent to baby hairs. Hello, receding hairline.

If you're like us, you'll start slicking your hair down in ways you never did before (with a toothbrush and hairspray), you'll experiment with new styles (exceptionally messy top knot), and you'll bitch to your partner, who will look you in the eye and tell you they honestly doesn't see any difference in your hair whatsoever. And then you will cry some more.

STAGE FOUR: REGROWTH

Just as you begin to make peace with the baldness, you'll look in the mirror one day and discover that those hairs that fell out last month are now being replaced by tiny new hairs. REGROWTH!
On the one hand, you're happy about it. On the other hand, you realize that the only thing more annoying than looking like you're prematurely balding is looking like you're wearing a spiky, frizz-hairband.

STAGE FIVE: CHANGE

You'll eventually come to terms with the fact that your hair isn't the hair it once was. Likewise, you're not the woman you once were. You're new and improved, and you better believe you're gonna make sure your hair is new and improved as well.

Off to the hairdresser you'll go. If they know you well, they'll be expecting you. Now is the time for fun. What's it going to be? Blunt bangs? A bob? A "lob"? The world is your oyster.

No matter what happens in that chair, accept the following two truths: First, whether or not you're loving what's happening north of your neck right now, you just scored at least an hour or two of precious alone time at the salon; and second, it's just hair.

You may not believe us right now, but one day this will all be over, and you'll be the veteran mom telling your unsuspecting pregnant friend to enjoy that shit while it lasts.

THE ALMIGHTY MOM

Ah, the Almighty Mom. We've all met her.

Her shit doesn't stink, and her offspring is a gifted, gorgeous, genius-baby who does the family taxes. She's the self-appointed authority on all things motherhood, and she became an expert in child-rearing the moment she got knocked up.

Before you had a kid, you could tolerate her. Now that you've got a child of your own, and she's sitting beside you on the couch preaching her sleep-training methods, you're searching for a wall to bang your head against.

The Almighty Mom particularly sucks because in your exhausted, dazed and confused, first-time mom brain, there's a chance you might actually take her seriously and feel like a shitty parent compared to her. Fuck that.

We're here to call these ladies out, because there isn't a mom in the world who has her shit together 100 percent of the time. Anyone who feels the need to brag in the presence of other mothers is just trying to draw attention away from her own insecurities. We promise, these moms also deal with non-Instagram-worthy drama, and they too sob in the middle of the day, just like the rest of us.

If you happen to be that mama who sometimes (perhaps inadvertently) goes on and on about how impeccable your motherhood experience has been, and how perfect and special your child is, think about being on the receiving end of that convo and how utterly annoying it sounds.

Not all moms want to spend an afternoon discussing nap schedules and poo consistency. There are more interesting things to talk about. Besides, who cares about who's doing it best? We're all doing the best we can, and that's all that matters.

So what should you do when an Almighty Mom parks herself across from you and unloads her unsolicited advice? Be kind. All that glory-talk is probably coming from a void that needs to be filled, so help a sister out. Listen, smile, nod, and say, "That's good to know. Thanks for the tip!"

Then do whatever the fuck you want anyway.

A NOTE FOR (NEW) REBEL PAPAS

Hey, Pops!

Congrats on the whole dad thing. Glad to have you on the team. If you've opened this book hoping to get some insight into The Secret Lives of Moms, welcome. Feel free to stay a while (at your own risk, of course).

Since you're here, there are a few things we need you to know about your new life.

The first few months on the job will likely be tough for you. You'll probably feel pretty useless at times, and you'll be unbelievably exhausted. We feel you, dude. But as you wade through the haze of the newborn days, remember that your lady is, at all times, at least 200 percent more exhausted than you are.

Her body is in overdrive. She's hyper-aware of your baby's every noise and movement. Her vagina feels like it's just gotten into a violent street-fight (or she's recovering from massive abdominal surgery - either way, OUCH), and her hormones are making her feel insane 24/7.

While this time in your life is undoubtedly scary and stressful, you need to realize that the brunt of this parenting gig is falling squarely on your lady's shoulders right now. If she's making it look easy, it's because she's a goddamn hero. It is not easy. She's busting her exhausted ass off to make sure she's doing right by your baby, so go tell her she's awesome (right now). She IS awesome, and she deserves to hear it.

With all that being said, we really are rooting for you to kill it in your new dad role, so here are a few insider tips to keep you out of the dog house for the next little while. Don't say we never do anything nice for you.

◊◊◊

DON'T PLAY DUMB

Early parenthood is a classic case of the blind leading the blind. Please do NOT excuse yourself from any activity pertaining to the baby (like changing shitty diapers or going to settle the baby at 3:00 a.m.) by citing the fact that your lady is "just so much better at it than me." Don't be that guy. You're better than that guy.

CONTROL YOUR LOINS

It's really hard to wait a whole six weeks (or more) for the recovery process to end. We get that. We also get that, despite how your lady may feel about her postpartum bod, you probably still find her irresistible (bless you). But the truth is, this time really isn't about you. It's about her and her recovery. Right now, her body needs time to heal, and if she's not ready, then fall in line, my friend. One day she will be ready, and trust us when we tell you that it will be worth the wait. In the meantime, follow her lead. When it's go time, you'll be the first to know.

PRACTICE SAYING "YES, DEAR"

Early parenthood is not the time to argue about the trivial details of everyday life. There's too much crazy shit happening, and everyone is beyond tired. This simple phrase, passed down through generations of men the world over, will literally save your ass.

ASK HOW YOU CAN HELP

If you find yourself feeling like a fish out of water, not knowing what to do to make postpartum life a little easier for your lady, just ask. Chances are, there are a million things you can do to help. Shit always needs to be sterilized, the house could always use vacuuming, and your baby-mama would probably give her left arm for thirty minutes alone in a hot shower. So hop to it! This is the kind of karma you want on your side.

BE PATIENT

This one isn't easy. Babies are really cute and sweet and snuggly, but several times a day, every day, they make you question your very existence. If you happen to be at home during "the witching hours" (yes, they have a name), STAY CALM. This is a great time to start practicing extreme patience. Let the baby cry for a minute while YOU figure out what it needs. Your girl spends all day, every day, trouble-shooting, and it's exhausting. If you can be a beacon of peace and calm during the times when everyone is about to lose their shit, you're going to come out looking like the goddamn Dali Lama.

Namaste and best of luck, Rebel Papa. You got this.

Part 3
ON BABIES

"Now the thing about having a baby – and I can't be the first person to have noticed this – is that thereafter you have it."

– Jean Kerr

UNSOLICITED RAPID-FIRE ADVICE

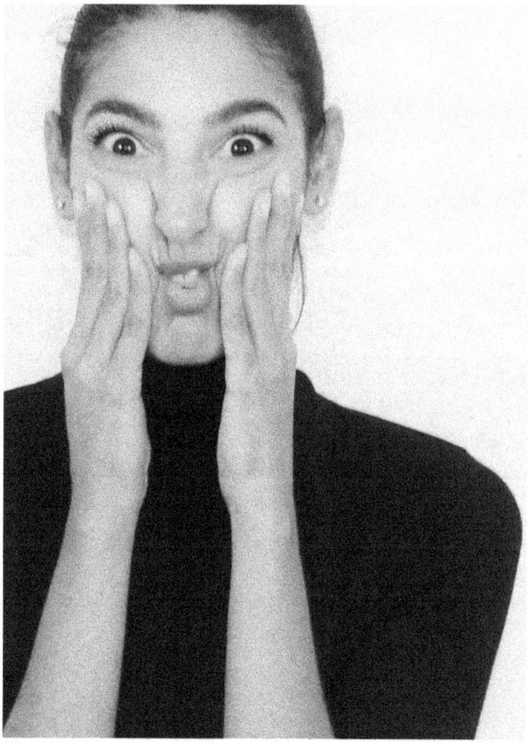

◊ Infants may be tiny and helpless, but they're also pretty indestructible. Don't let them freak you out.

◊ Don't be alarmed by weird skin things. Babies are strange and so is baby skin. Nine times out of ten, it's nothing.

◊ Cure cradle cap by applying a hefty dose of coconut or olive oil to your baby's head and popping a little cotton hat over the whole mess. Leave it on for ten minutes, remove the hat, and then gently remove the softened scalp flakes (ew) with a fine baby-comb.

◊ Don't rush your baby into crawling or walking. Trust us, you will miss the immobility when it's gone.

◊ There's no need to baby-proof your entire house; just teach them not to touch your shit. It's tedious, but then you can bring them to other people's houses one day, and they'll know what *the look* means.

◊ As long as your baby is happy and safe, there's no need to rush to their crib when they wake up in the morning or after naps. If your kid wakes up screaming bloody murder, go get them. But if they're chillin', then just let chillin' babies chill.

◊ Learn how to give yourself a quick and easy up-do (slicked back into a ponytail or tossed into a messy bun). Lucky for you, greasy hair is great for styling.

◊ Don't underestimate the healing power of breast milk. Rashes, weird eye things, scrapes and cuts - when in doubt, squirt some milk on it and watch the magic unfold.

◊ Make it a point to get out of the house without your tiny ball and chain every so often. Even if it's just to go back to the pharmacy. Again.

◊ It's okay to let your baby get a little dirty, and it's fine if they eat random stuff off the ground (excluding the obvious shit). Hello, strong immune system!

◊ Nothing with babies is permanent. Whenever you're about to lose it, just remember: IT'S A PHASE. Phases end. We promise.

◊ Use your baby's wet wipes as makeup removal wipes. Models use them on set; why shouldn't you?

◊ Fill your thermos with an adult beverage for that mid-summer 7:00 p.m. stroll. No one will ever know.

THE MOST SURPRISING THING ABOUT THE NEWBORN PHASE

We both spent the first twenty-four hours after our babies were born doing the same stuff every modern mom in the Western World does: requesting WIFI passwords and pain killers, wishing the hospital was equipped with *proper* coffee, and marveling at the absolute perfection of the little beings that just emerged from our bodies.

The only thought running through our minds that first day was "this is the best." This baby is the best. This baby is so chill. This baby is so cute. I'm a fucking rock star. Our lives are going to be so awesome. I'm going to be the best mom ever. This rules.

Then night two rolled around, and with it the first of many surprises: cluster feeding.

In case you're not yet familiar with the term, it's something newborns do when the satiation from the womb wears off about twenty-four hours after birth, and they suddenly transform into starving velociraptors who demand milk every hour, on the hour. All. Night. Long.

Neither of us will ever forget that fateful first cluster feed. It felt like the baby was playing a cruel joke on us, like "Hey, I know you're currently recovering from major abdominal surgery, but would you mind just staying up all night while I try to extract milk from your tender breasts, even though you don't know what you're doing and it's going to hurt like a bitch? Awesome, thanks."

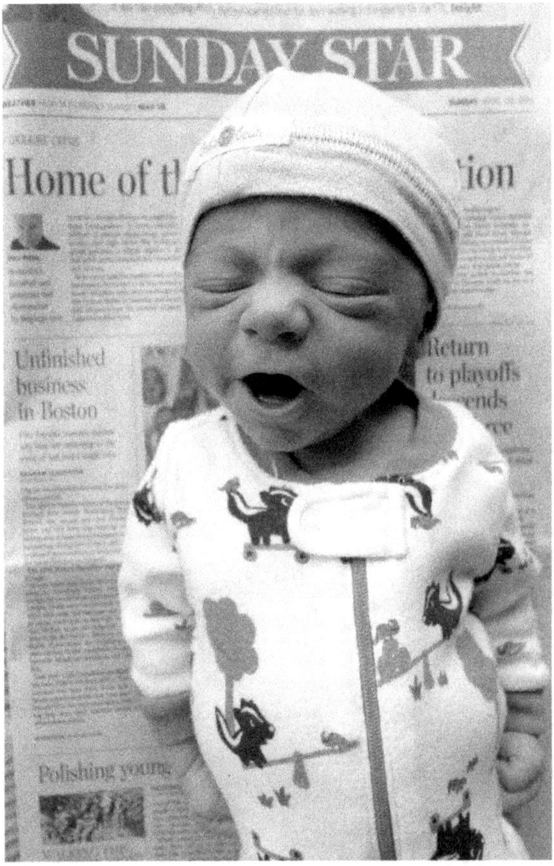

The surprises only multiplied and intensified in the days that followed.

Surprise! The baby hates being put down.

Surprise! The baby shits fifty times a day (fine, not fifty, but definitely ten, which is still way more than we were expecting from a tiny baby).

Surprise! The baby can't deal with your milk let down, so he chokes every time you try to get him to latch.

Surprise! The baby has day and night mixed up, so he snoozes from 8:00 a.m. to 9:00 p.m. and then parties from 10:00 p.m. to 7:00 a.m.

Surprise! The baby hates that $300 designer bouncy chair you bought him.

Surprise! The baby loves that hideous $30 colourful monstrosity of a chair that your mother-in-law bought him.

Surprise! The baby has a case of acne that rivals your 13-year-old nephew (and there's nothing you can do about it other than wait it out).

Surprise! The baby hates his car seat. And his stroller. And his bassinet.

Surprise! The baby has to go to a hundred doctor's appointments in his first twelve weeks of life (fine, not a hundred, but at least five, which is still way more than we were expecting for a tiny baby).

Surprise! The baby vomits so forcefully that it hits the wall behind you (and the sofa, and the chair, and the dog, and his clothes, and your clothes).

Surprise! The baby cries every day from 5:00 p.m. to 8:00 p.m., for no reason. #WitchingHour

Can you make it through this onslaught of surprises while (a) simultaneously recovering from the most intense physical trauma you've ever endured, (b) trying to function on two hours of sleep a night, and (c) dealing with insane postpartum hormones?

Surprise! Yes, you can. You're a mom now, and you are officially tough as shit. Welcome to the other side.

Story-time with Nikita('s Grandma)

WHAT A (GREAT) GRANDMA WANTS YOU TO KNOW ABOUT INFANTS

My maternal grandmother, whom we call Oma, is 85-years-old and quick as a whip. She is a mother of three, a grandmother of eight, and a great-grandmother of five (so far). Not only has she had a hand in raising each and every one of us (yes, all sixteen!), but she loves babies so much that she decided to spend a big chunk of her retirement working at a daycare, specializing in infant care for babies aged three months to one year.

The woman is an oracle. I could not have written a book about anything baby-related without including the best advice she has ever given me about newborns:

Have patience with your newborn, because this is all newer to him than it is to you. He's never felt air on his skin, and he's never heard the sounds of the outside world like this before. He's scared and he's sad, because he just left the only world he's ever known. The only thing he recognizes here is you, your voice, your movements, and your smell. You are still his home.

So when he cries for you in the night, don't be vex with him.* When he wants to be held all day, don't get frustrated. When he won't let anyone else comfort him, don't be upset.

Just help him get through this tough phase in his life. Soon everything will become more familiar to him, and he will get accustomed to his life in this new world. But for now, just be there for him. The time for schedules and rules will come, but this is not it. Now is a time to enjoy.

So, go - enjoy your baby. No guilt, no fear, no apologies.
Oma said so.

**Yes, my grandma is Jamaican.*

THE GREAT (RIDICULOUS) FORMULA DEBATE

We've always found the whole Breast vs. Formula debate to be one of the more infuriating points of contention within the parenting community. How to feed your child is a deeply personal decision for any family to make. Anyone with Internet access knows that the benefits of breastfeeding are endless. Sure, breast is often best ... but what about when it's not?

In many circumstances, breastfeeding (or attempting to breastfeed) causes more stress to either mama or baby (or both) than it's worth. Some women straight up can't do it for physical or medical reasons, no matter how many lactation consultants you throw their way. Knowing that, shouldn't we all – despite our various beliefs on the topic - stay the hell out of it and trust individual mothers' decision-making abilities? Don't we all deserve a little more credit than we give each other?

Yeah. We do.

JETSET BABY

No matter how terrifying this prospect may seem, the best time to travel with your child is when they're between zero and six-months old. They're immobile, they sleep a lot, and there's literally nothing a boob (or pacifier) can't fix. Most importantly, they're not relying on constant entertainment, meaning you can chill out and actually enjoy your time away.

Will your babe go buck-wild and cry for an entire flight? Maybe. But know this: millions of babies have cried on millions of flights before you, and no one remembers. If it happens, just try to calm your spawn and get over it. Earbuds and movies are available on planes for a reason.

Let's move away from the things you can't control, and focus on what you can.

Pro Tips:

- Travel in a pack. The more hands on deck, the smoother the whole experience will be. Grandparents, aunties, and friends make excellent on-the-road babysitters.

- Don't skimp on diapers. You never know when a three-diaper-poo-explosion is just around the corner.

- Start packing a week before your trip. It's going to feel like you're bringing the whole damn house, and in a way, you are. Not attempting to do it all the night before will keep anxiety levels at bay.

- Don't expect special treatment. If your kid falls asleep in the stroller in line to go through security, you're still going to have to take him out to go through the metal detectors (and he will wake up). Don't panic. Just roll with the punches; the whole ordeal will be over soon.

- Bring your baby carrier. It frees up your hands while you're navigating through the airport, and may even allow you to flip through a magazine if your baby conks out on the flight.

- Don't bother pre-boarding. Yes, it may be tempting to get in and get settled, but the less time spent on the plane, the better.

- Smile a lot at surrounding passengers. If you're nice to them, they'll be more likely to engage in a game of peek-a-boo (or hand you back whatever toy was launched in their direction).

- Fight the urge to bring special "care packages" for people on the plane. This trend is bullshit. Crying kids on a plane is a reality of travelling, and everyone needs to get the fuck over it.

- Don't worry about liquid restrictions. They will let you bring all kinds of milk and water on board as long as it's for the baby.

- Do not forget the snacks. Load up your diaper bag with finger foods that will keep your little one occupied. Mum Mums, blueberries, grapes, steamed carrot sticks, crackers, cheese - pile it all in.

- Purchase a seat for your baby (if it's not way out of budget). This way, you will be able to bring your car seat on board and strap them in, making them more comfortable, and therefore more likely to sleep during the flight.

- Don't rush yourself. Pre-baby travel was easy. You used to be able to just grab your passport and credit card and show up sixty minutes before departure. That is no longer your reality. Be organized and leave early. Give yourself plenty of time for emergency diaper changes, impromptu feedings, and properly checking in your eighteen bags.

- Bring a change of clothes for yourself in your carry-on. Something is inevitably going to get smeared or barfed or spilled all over you in flight, and sitting in it for hours isn't the sexiest.

Bonus travel tips for non-infants *(ahem, good luck):*

Once your little one becomes more mobile (somewhere around twelve to eighteen months), you're slightly more fucked. A three-hour flight can feel transcontinental if you're not prepared for the worst.

We wouldn't want you to be ill-equipped for an excursion with a more active spawn, so we've compiled some additional travel tips that will have you worrying about one thing and one thing only: what kind of vino is available 30,000 feet in the air.

- (Wo)man up and go through the Global Entry application process. This VIP access will save you hours in lines and ensure your sanity doesn't get left behind at customs when your toddler suddenly loses the ability to use their legs.

- Book flights around their nap schedule. If you can get them snoozing during the flight, it'll shave off an hour or two of entertainment. On the other hand, if you know your kid will *not* nap if she doesn't have a bed in which to do so, then shoot for a morning flight—she'll nap upon arrival and won't be a total a-hole at dinner that night.

- Bring books. Lots and lots of books (if they like books, of course). Bonus tip: buy the light-weight, fabric kind to save your shoulders from a heavy carry-on.

- Don't forget familiar sleeping cues like blankies, soothers, and anything else that smells like home. This will ease them into sleep mode with less drama.

- Factor in delays and stay away from late flights, because you know an overtired toddler gives zero fucks about unforeseen circumstances, regardless of how many trips to the gift store you make.

- Don't over pack your carry-on with toys. Bring the top five faves and a few different activity options. Let's be real, a jacked-up iPad with three seasons of whatever the hell they're into right now will likely be the winner anyway. Bonus Tip: Download some educational games; it'll keep them busy AND you'll feel bad-ass when they recite the alphabet perfectly.

- Wear breathable, comfy clothes that can endure toddler abuse. They can (and will) treat your body like a rock-climbing wall, and high-waisted raw denim will not help your cause. Assuming you'd like to be comfortable without feeling like a total slob, choose loose, soft, dark clothes.

- Get to the airport with plenty of time to spare, so it seems more like a playful and fun adventure and less like *The Amazing Race*. Murphy's Law always applies to rushed situations - do not play with fire.

- Bring a light-weight umbrella stroller if your kid frequently has ants in her pants. It'll keep her trapped, so you don't appear to be the frazzled mother you actually are.

- Do yourself a solid and pee before you board, even if you have to force it. There's a good chance you won't be moving for a while, and a twenty-six-pound, hot and sweaty kid is the last thing you need on your full bladder.

- Baby wipes should be within reach at all times. Besides cleaning your child and all the surface areas at the airport / in the airplane, they will also keep your skin glowing throughout the whole ordeal.

- Diaper-bag essentials: teething remedies, allergy medicine, fever medicine, Polysporin, cold and cough syrup, Band-Aids, Q-Tips, bug spray, after-bite, and a thermometer. Throw in some rose-water spray for yourself as an in-flight refresher that will have people wondering how in the hell you're keeping so well.

In summary, if you were an avid traveler before, there's no reason you can't be one now! Is it a pain in the ass? Kind of. Is it worth the trouble? Absolutely. The memories you make during family vacations will stay with all of you forever, and instilling a love of travel in your child from a young age is a gift they will thank you for a million times over in the future.

GET YOUR SLEEP (TRAINING) ON

There are a lot of you out there who don't believe in sleep training, and that's fine. Go on with your bad selves, mamas (and feel free to skip ahead to the next chapter). Having said that, we also know that there are equally as many of you who are done feeling like lactating zombies and are desperate to feel like actual (sleeping) human beings again. If you fall into the latter category, and you're hell-bent on teaching your kid how to sleep without losing your mind in the process, we can help you out with some tips.

For us, sleep is non-negotiable. We are not - nor have we ever been - the kind of people who can even pretend to have our shit together on four hours of sleep. For the first few months of our kids' lives, we felt like hell. We were tired all the time. We were grumpy. Our appetites were a mess. We were nowhere near our best selves.

As soon as we taught our spawn to fall asleep on their own without nursing, pacing, bouncing, swaying, lunging, or shushing, they were noticeably happier. And you know who else was happier? US! WE WERE HAPPIER!

Once we were sleeping through the night again, we felt like better, more patient moms. Moms who had a chance to recharge their batteries. Moms who were able to take on the daily grind without crying in line at the coffee shop.

If that's what you need in your life, then sleep training might be worth a try. Is it easy? No. Is anything easy when it comes to babies? We'll let you answer that one for yourself.

Now let's get you through the initial shittiness so that you can reclaim those Zs (and your sanity) ASAP, shall we?

- Get your doctor involved, even just for peace of mind. Any time after baby's four-month checkup, ask your doctor if they think baby is getting enough calories during the day to hold her over at night. Knowing that your kid is not waking due to hunger will make it easier not to run to her offering a boob whenever she squawks in the middle of the night.

- For some reason, babies seem to have their best sleep when they go to bed at 6:30 p.m. It seems insanely early, but if you're going to give sleep training a try, starting with an early bed-time can make life a lot easier.

- Put baby down when she's tired (but not losing-her-shit, wanted-to-go-to-bed-five-hours-ago tired). Google "infant sleep cues". Watch her like a hawk. When you see a yawn or an eye rub, it's go time.

- Once you identify when your baby is sleepy, track her rhythm. Kids are pretty consistent with wake times. When they are really tiny (around four to six months), they can only function with two-hour (max) wake-windows. At six to twelve months, that stretches to three-hour wake-windows, and thereafter, four to five-hour wake-windows (at which point they're down to one nap). Tracking it like this is much easier than trying to get them on a strict time schedule.

- Develop a sleep cue from you to your baby. It doesn't have to be a big, elaborate series of events (i.e. three books, two songs, a bath, a massage, a story, a bottle, and bed). It just needs to be something you do to tell baby that it's bed-time. For example, you could try singing "Twinkle, Twinkle Little Star" on the way up the stairs. Any other trip upstairs is not accompanied by a tune. When there is singing involved, your baby will know it's time to shut it down. If your kid is still an infant, you may feel like an asshole putting on a show for a little seal who shows no sign of computing, but trust us, if you do it every time, they start to clue in faster than you'd think.

- In the beginning (i.e. the first week of sleep training), try doing something loud and productive right when you put the baby down. Not only will it drown out the crying so you don't feel like bolting up to baby's room every fifteen seconds, but it will also help you pass the time more quickly (ten minutes can feel like an eternity when you're sitting outside of your baby's door, weeping as she shrieks, but not so much of an eternity when you finally get your main floor vacuumed). Another huge benefit of the "noisy chore" trick is that it serves as a reminder that, if you stick with this sleep-training thing, you will once again be able to get shit done. You'll finally have some GD "me time" again, from 6:30 p.m. until your own bed-time! After you've spent 24/7 with a baby attached to your body for nearly half a year, trust us, it feels really friggin' good.

- Don't create an unrealistic sleep environment. Make sure you can more or less recreate the experience of going to sleep for baby with minimal effort if you're not at home. Most kids can sleep with a bit of light (curtains, but not black-out curtains), a crib, a blankie, and a noise machine. Most can also sleep with you living your life around them (read: watching TV, entertaining guests, and other loud adult things). Anytime you're at someone else's house or out-of-town, this situation can be recreated with a pack'n'play, standard window coverings, a white noise app on your smart phone, and their little blankie from home.

- When the baby inevitably wakes up in the night, always give them ten minutes to figure their shit out before going in to intervene. Most of the time, they won't make it to ten minutes before falling back asleep. If they do, it's boob (or soother) and right back to bed. At the very beginning, if they wake up three times, maybe one of those times will last long enough to prompt you to get up and feed them. Dealing with one wake up between 6:30 p.m. and 7:00 a.m. will feel a lot more reasonable than that every-two-hours-all-night-long crap.

- Sleep train for naps using a similar tactic. If they have a short, shitty nap, give them ten minutes in the crib when they wake up to see if they'll go back to sleep. You'll be surprised at how often they'll conk back out for an additional hour.

- Take regressions in stride. Every new skill (and bout of sickness) can be a setback, from sitting, to crawling, to talking, to standing, to teething, to colds, to growth spurts, etc. You know you're in one when there's literally a random overnight shift in sleeping patterns (i.e. nights that make you wake up in the morning thinking your life is over and you'll never sleep again). You can get through regressions by reminding yourself that all is not lost and this is just a phase. During these phases, though, you just have to go full on survival mode. Nursing, soothers, bottles, cuddles - WHATEVER. Once it starts to let up (longer stretches between waking up at night), go back into sleep-training mode.

- Have your partner go comfort the baby if she's inconsolable in the night. If you go (especially if you're nursing), baby will lose her shit until you cave and feed her because she KNOWS it's there. Kids always give up faster with dad / a non-nursing parent. Go figure.

- If you do cave and end up feeding your crying cherub (happens to the best of us), don't panic and pick her right back up again if she cries as soon as you lay her back down. Leave the room calmly, and give her ten minutes before sending your partner in to comfort her.

- Don't let sleep training make you crazy. This process is ongoing, and it's frustrating AF. Some nights it'll be a total breeze, other nights you'll spend 6:30 p.m. till 11:00 p.m. going back and forth from the nursery to the sofa with a baby who just really doesn't feel like going to bed. Whatever. When that happens, our policy is that as long as it isn't creating a new trend, who cares? Don't be hard on yourself about any of it- no need to make a high-stress situation more stressful.

MOM INSOMNIA DEBUNKED

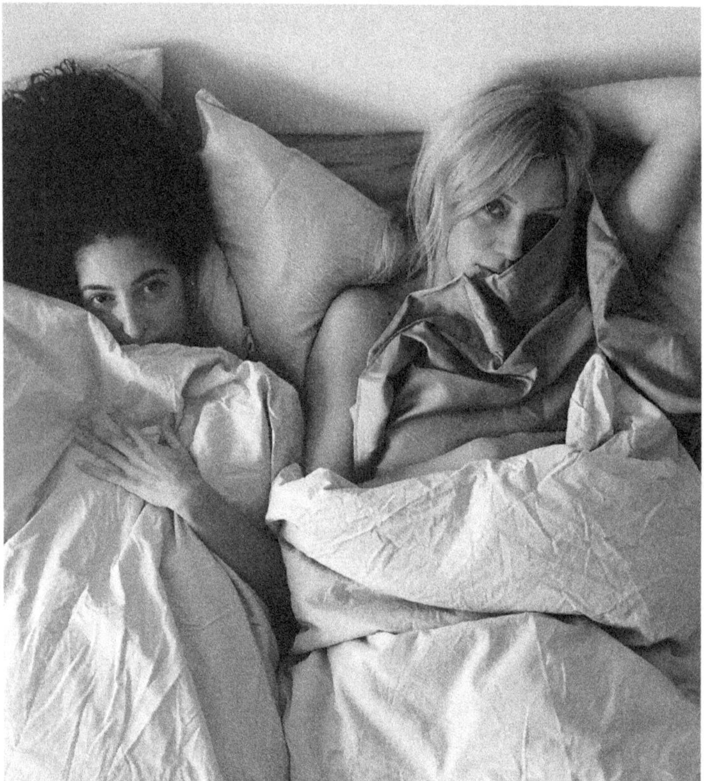

The following happens to about 99 percent of new moms: one day, you wake up at 7:00 a.m. and realize that your baby has slept through the night. You think this must be a fluke, but then she does it again on the second night, and then every night after that for a week. You finally allow yourself to accept the sweet truth: OMG, MY BABY IS SLEEPING LIKE A REGULAR HUMAN.

Your first thought is that you've finally made it to the other side. After months of getting no sleep yourself, you're about to get back on track and sleep through the night again, just like your sweet babe.

That night, you put junior to sleep and settle into your own bed, ready to get the rest you deserve, only to be up until the wee hours of the morning over-thinking improbable scenarios, scrolling through social-media accounts in Australia, and researching insomnia while silently sobbing inside.

WHYYYYYYY!! you think. *Why can't I fall asleep?? Why must I be punished when I am so desperately in need of rest?! AND WHY IS MY PARTNER SNORING LIKE AN ASSHOLE?!*

We know, babe. We've all been there, and it sucks. It sucks almost as much as the people who tell you to "nap when the baby naps."

If you're suffering from mom-insomnia, you've probably tried all the classic remedies: sleepy herbal teas, all-natural sleep sprays, melatonin, magnesium, calcium, Tylenol PM, NyQuil, Benadryl, yoga, meditation, books, baths, less screen time, more red wine, weed, sex (side note: that only works for men), and so on and so forth.

Here are some Rebel-approved tips to get some much-needed Zs:

- Keep the screen of the baby monitor off, and the sound on low. When your kid wails, you'll hear it, and if they squeak, you won't even notice. Voilà.

- Take any thoughts that keep you up and redirect them to something else. Try mentally planning your over-the-top birthday party instead. What are you going to wear? What's the theme? Who will you invite? *Cue drowsiness*

- Set a hard bedtime for yourself and honour it. Choose a reasonable hour, and when the clock strikes, stop everything you're doing and get your ass to bed. No excuses.

- Lower your overall caffeine intake. Attempt the impossible and have one (yes, one) coffee a day, preferably before noon so the caffeine has time to escape your body by bedtime. If you want to be a total bad-ass, have hot water with lemon and cayenne in the morning for a massive boost to your energy (and metabolism - YAY).

- Don't exercise an hour or two before bed as it can keep you wired. (If you want to be a total keener, don't exercise at all.)

- Turn off ALL screens at least an hour before bed. As much as your thumbs may be twitching to check Instagram one last time, it's worth the FOMO to get some rest. Leave your laptop and phone charging in another room, and keep some good books on your bedside table.

- Create a bedtime routine for yourself and treat it just as seriously as your baby's. This will take some commitment, because most days you'll be too damn lazy to follow through. You have to remind yourself how valuable sleep is. Example: Drink some decaf tea (or warm milk with honey) and read for half an hour. Hell, throw in a bath if that's your thing.

- Look into the magical powers of Turmeric. In powder form, capsule form, or prepared as a tea, this natural ingredient has been said to greatly improve sleep for those with insomnia and sleep disorders. Google it.

- Try acupuncture and Chinese Medicine (aka herbal teas). Most people assume that these practices have more to do with physical pain relief, but they also help to regulate your system from within. This duo has been known to tackle menstrual pain, fertility problems, stress, and anxiety. Google that one, too.

- Borrow your baby's noise machine. Many people swear by being lulled gently to sleep by a steady stream of spring water (or good old-fashioned white noise), as it naturally helps you to wind down, and stops your mind from wandering.

- Switch the monitor to your partner's side and put them in charge of standing guard at night. This way, you can rest easy knowing that, if the baby cries, SOMEONE ELSE will hear it.

- Speaking of partners, if yours is snoring up a storm, get them the hell out. You'll be surprised how well a private sleep sanctuary can work. If you happen to have a guest room, BINGO, my friend. Use it.

- Keep your room temperature slightly on the cool side. There is a direct relationship between body temperature and sleep. If your room is too hot, it may make you restless.

With that, we bid you a good night. May you dream of John Stamos.

YOU'RE ALLOWED TO SAY "THIS SUCKS"

Just so you know, as we speak, there are thousands - likely hundreds of thousands - of women out there chugging back wine, smoking flower, taking up yoga / hiking / meditating / whatever, just to cope with the fact that sometimes, having a baby totally sucks.

We're not saying that all mothers feel this way. It would be crazy to assume that every woman has the exact same experience of early motherhood (RIGHT?). But a lot of moms *do* feel this way. Maybe you feel this way.

Why are we willing to accept women talking openly about their "coping mechanisms," yet people lose their GD minds the minute a woman comes out and admits the truth about the thing she's actually trying to cope with? Why are we so shocked when women admit their not-so-secret desire to flee from their role as "mom" for a hot minute?

The sleep deprivation, the constant feeling that you're "not doing it right," and the pressure from outside sources to "enjoy every minute" is a lot to handle.

Some people adjust to their new lives faster than others, and in time, we all adjust (yes, even us mommy-group drop-outs). But if you're having a rough time right now, you are fully allowed to say, "this fucking sucks." When you've got young children, that's a completely justifiable statement.

Unfortunately, a lot of women face harsh criticism or are written off as terrible mothers as soon as they attempt to open up about any negative feelings they have about motherhood. That makes zero sense.

What these brave women deserve is respect for their honesty, and support to continue being loving parents to their children. Does it not make more sense to listen to a woman in distress, rather than try to silence her?

So, Mama, whenever you feel inclined to do so, please openly declare, "This fucking sucks." Do whatever you can to create safe spaces for your fellow mamas wherein *they* feel as though *they* can say, "This fucking sucks," too. The only way we can hope to find meaningful solutions to our collective problems is to be given the grace to admit that they exist in the first place.

LESSONS FROM A SIX-MONTH-OLD

You will learn a lot from your children, especially when you take a step back and take a look at the world through their eyes. Here are some valuable life lessons we've learned from our own babies. Feel free to generously apply them to your daily life.

◊◊◊

Persistence is a powerful tool. Pursue your goals and dreams with the same level of commitment that a baby applies when attempting to open (and empty) all the drawers and cabinets in your kitchen.

Getting excited about a new day (every day) sets the tone for life. A baby almost always wakes up with a smile, pumped to practice new skills and learn new tricks. You should do the same.

Don't like something? Toss it. Remember that time Grandma came over with a gift that your baby wasn't interested in? BOOM- thrown to the wayside, without thinking twice about it. Use this definitive de-cluttering technique in your own life, but with a slightly more adult level of tact.

Want something? Go get it! Opportunities exist to be seized. If it's important, go for it like a baby goes for a cookie that fell on the ground.

Don't knock it 'til you try it. You don't necessarily need to try eating the blades of grass in your backyard (leave that to junior), but let your baby's penchant for trying new things inspire you to get out of your comfort zone; you'll be a better woman for it.

Be selective with who you let into your personal space. Have you ever seen a baby react to someone with questionable energy? Not everyone is worth your time. It's totally cool (and necessary) to wisely choose with whom you surround yourself.

People-watching is an art. Babies learn from carefully studying the folks around them. You would be amazed at what you too can learn by following suit. Don't stare, though. It's awkward.

When you fall, pick yourself back up and start over. Babies practice this important skill a million times a day. It's called resilience, and we're all born with it. If you've lost it, rediscover it. If you've got it, hang on to it for dear life.

Subtle flirting can really get you places. Babies get away with everything, just by flashing a sweet smile or batting their pretty little eyes. Adopt this tactic to accomplish anything from getting out of a speeding ticket to encouraging your partner to take out the trash.

When all else fails, bust out the waterworks. Make like a baby and open those hormonal floodgates when you really want to get your way. It works (almost) every time.

MUSH 101

While introducing solids is both rewarding and hilarious, be warned: It's a lot more fun in theory than it is in reality. Be prepared to clean sticky rice off the floor and rinse yogourt out of your hair three times a day for the next little while.

First things first: Doctor's orders change as often as fashion trends, so the recommendations you receive today may be a distant memory by next season. With that in mind, start slow. Trust your chosen physician and your tiger-mama instincts. This stage should be (at least moderately) enjoyable, so don't let it turn you into an anxiety-filled baby-food freak.

If you're a keener, rest assured that there are plenty of books out there with a plethora of ideas for your new dining guest. For the rest of us, make a quick list of basics to start with. Steam them, mush them up, and ta-da! Baby food.

Here are a few professional (if we do say so ourselves) life hacks for solids:

- Invest in an all-in-one steamer / blender contraption (check your local baby store). You'll use it 'round the clock, and it travels easily. Stove-top drama is a thing of the past! Shout out to modern technology.

- Your baby will love certain things one week and hate them the next, or vice versa. Don't worry about it, but remember to never make too much of any one thing at a time; it will just result in a shit ton of wasted food. Buy less, and get in the habit of making smaller portions.

- Ice-cube trays are perfect for portion control. Blend up some mush, pour it into trays, freeze it, then transfer those frozen bad boys into a giant freezer bag and warm them up as needed. Start with half a cube at the beginning, then work up to one, two, three, and so on. Mix and match them for added variety.

- Start with veggies before moving on to fruit. If you were offered dessert first, wouldn't you say 'to hell with dinner'? Get the more unappealing foods happening early, and you'll be humble bragging about your toddler eating raw kale before you know it.

- Buy whatever is in season (extra points for local produce); it will keep you from falling into a food rut and force you to think of some new interesting combos to try on your little guinea pigs.

- Don't automatically assume your spawn will hate something. Babies don't know spinach is healthy and gross until you tell them so.

- Don't shy away from spices. Curry, dill, garlic, and yes, even a little salt and sugar will keep them interested and ready to be future foodies.

- As the weeks pass, make their food slightly chunkier until they are full-blown texture pros. It won't be long before they can chomp on baby pasta and baked goods with their little gums. Finally, a purpose for all those rotten bananas.

- Making smoothies is a lifesaver. It's an easy way to get your babe to try pretty much anything that can be sucked up through a straw. You can sneak in super foods like kale, blueberries, acai, cacao, lentils, broccoli, avocados, prunes, and anything else your heart desires. Sweeten things up with dates, mangos, or bananas if you're going heavy on the greens.

Our biggest piece of advice is to keep this whole experience a positive one. Don't get frustrated if on Monday your kid gladly eats an avocado, and by Tuesday it's the most horrifying thing you could possibly offer. Patience is the key ingredient when feeding babies.

There will also be days when your child will barely eat at all - days where you will wonder how in the hell he survived twelve hours on half a croissant and two raspberries. Let it go. Tomorrow is another day. It's almost impossible to starve your child at this age. You will know (insert screeching sound here) when they are hungry.

One last thing: allergies. The rules around all the things your babe is not allowed to come near can be daunting. The most recent recommendations say to expose your little ones to the scary potential allergens (peanuts, eggs, shellfish, etc.) sooner rather than later to avoid developing allergies in the first place; it worked for us. Test a small amount on their skin before feeding it to them to see if there are any alarming reactions, then start with super-small quantities, and work your way up over time.

**Reminder: We are not medically trained professionals! All of the above is simply what worked for us. Don't sue us if something doesn't work out, k? Always talk to your doctor first. (For a refresher on the topic, revert to xiv).*

GETTING STARTED:

Things you will need:

- *A fork (for mashing)*
- *A blender*
- *An awesome steam + blend system (bonus)*
- *Lots of bibs*
- *Patience*
- *Fine wine (for you, not them)*

FIRST MENU IDEAS:

- *Avocado and Banana / Mashed*
- *Sweet potatoes with butter, garlic, and dill / Cooked and mashed*
- *Lentils with lime / Cooked and pureed*
- *Carrot and apple / Steamed and pureed*
- *Warm cereal (rice, oatmeal, barley) with mashed or blended fruit*
- *Apricots and plums / Slow-cooked and pureed*
- *Peach and zucchini / Steamed and pureed*
- *Pear, parsnip, and kale / Steamed and pureed*
- *Apples with cinnamon / Steamed and pureed*
- *Pureed meats and low-mercury fish*
- *Yogurt with homemade unsweetened "jam"*

BONUS TIPS:

- Expect a mess. Don't be a rookie and serve pureed cherries over a white-shag carpet.

- In the beginning, you're just introducing food for fun. It's more of a taste test than a culinary experience. Keep the breast milk / formula going strong until your doctor tells you otherwise.

- When something works, jot it down. Make a list of breakfast, lunch, and dinner ideas that you can refer to. It's easy to get into a cycle of making the same stuff over and over, and that's boring.

- There are lots of great store-bought mush options these days. Buying the organic stuff will probably make you feel less guilty (worked for us), and these little pouches of love are great to have on hand for busy days on the go and any time you're travelling or away from home.

MOM-DATING: A GUIDE

If you're lucky enough to already have some cool mom friends, fantastic. If you don't currently have a like-minded partner in crime in your life, here's our checklist of qualities to look for in The One.

- She lets the F-Bomb slip at the playground in front of her toddler (and yours), and doesn't bat an eyelash.

- Her style resonates with you, and you secretly covet her sunglasses.

- Her youngster is in neutrals and/or non-offensive primary colours.

- She's on the playground bench, involved in leisurely phone-scrolling, with no desire to move - not because she's careless, but because she knows the value of space and independent play.

- She gives her babe a sip of her iced Americano after he incessantly begs for it, and knows that one sip won't kill him. She chooses her battles wisely and doesn't really care what anyone thinks.

- Her tone and volume are always calm and low. This classy babe clearly avoids drama.

- Her makeup is minimal, but she's somehow still effortlessly pulled together. You suspect she recently sprayed rose water on her face.

- She brought her kid to brunch, is drowning in mimosas, and gives no thought to the 25-year-old hipster who's offended by the animal-cookie crumbs all over the floor.

- She lets out a sigh when her cub throws a tantrum, sticks to her guns, and doesn't frantically stoop to their level. She speaks through clenched teeth and leaves if she must.

- You overhear her saying, "Whatever, if he doesn't nap, he'll just go to bed early." Any sign of chill is a good sign.

- She makes a sarcastic comment in your direction, "Now if only we could train them to make a good Martini…"

- You're pretty sure she has an actual martini in her kid's sippy cup.

It's a major blessing to have an ally in the trenches of motherhood who is transparent, empathetic, tough as nails, and is not a man. She will not judge you, pressure you, or lie to you about what this gig truly entails. She will always have your back, and together you will tackle this shit storm called parenting.

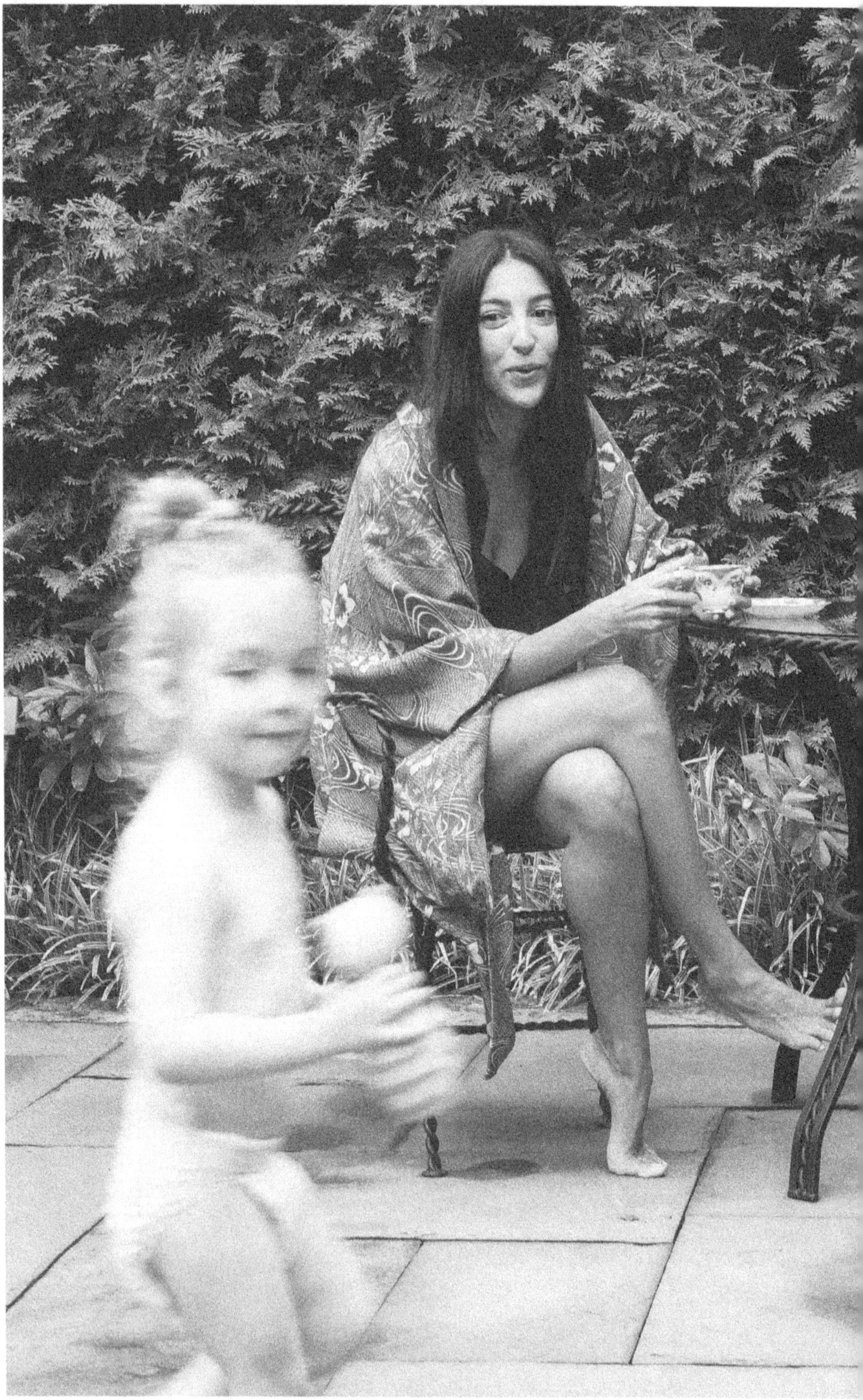

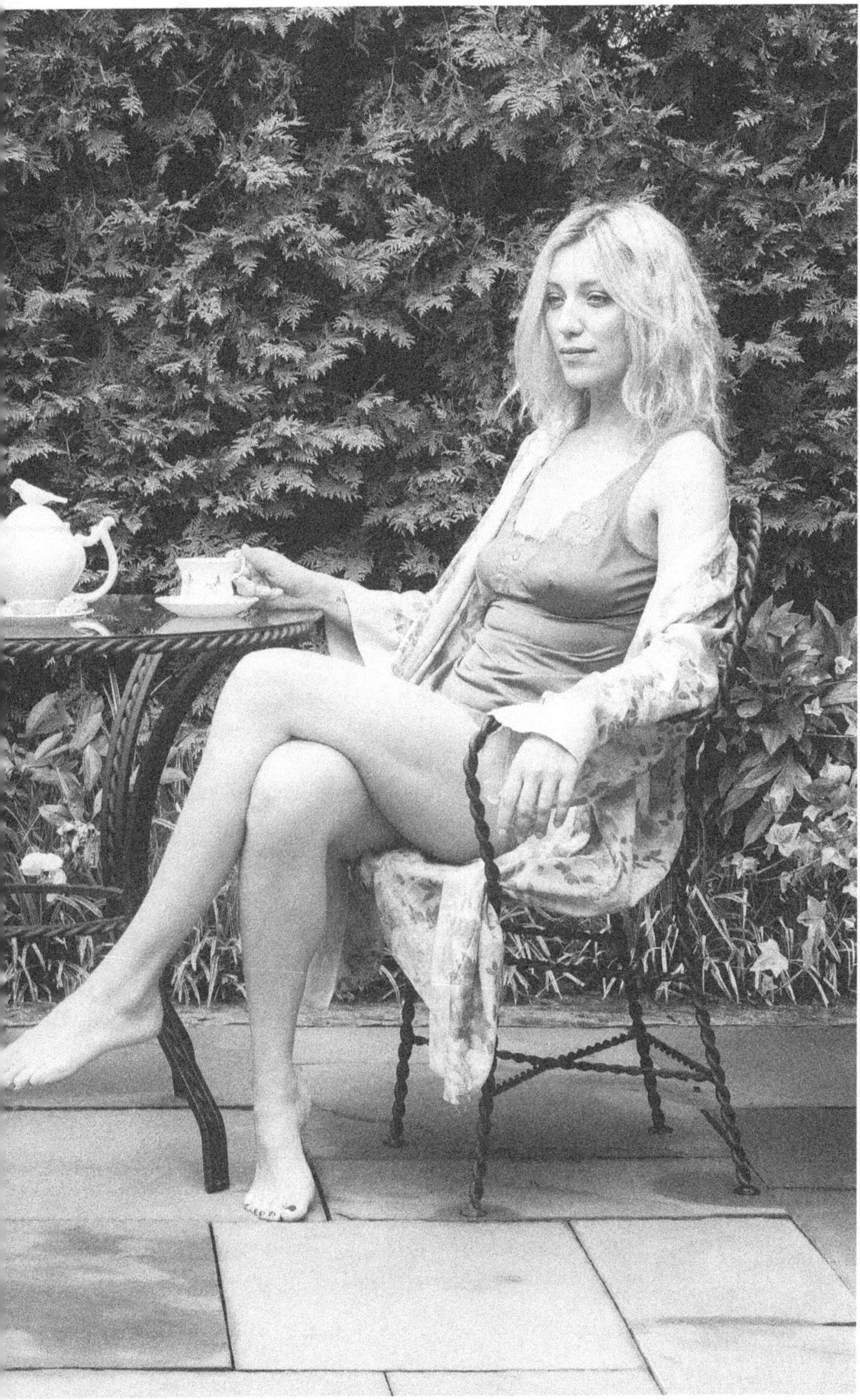

TEN PEOPLE YOUR BABY WILL MAKE YOU HATE

1. People who make plans to come over and show up late

They ask what time works for you; you say noon. At noon, the baby is up and the house is clean and you've had enough coffee to deal with life. Then they show up at two, when the baby is napping, there's Tupperware strewn about, and you're hitting your mid-day slump. Awesome, we should do this again soon.

2. People who put out cigarettes in parks

You know who loves picking up everything off the ground? BABIES. You know who puts everything they pick up in their mouths? BABIES.

3. Mid-day delivery people

Why must you knock SO LOUDLY? Do you think these modest row houses are secretly mansions, and we can't hear you because we're in the west wing? Please, for the love of naps, just knock gently.

4. Evening solicitors

We're not joining the church, we don't need you to check the furnace, and we're not interested in your chocolate-covered almonds. We cannot understand why you are banging on our doors at 9:00 p.m. when our babies are sleeping. Go home.

5. People who put their garbage cans in the middle of the sidewalk on garbage day

Thanks, bud. There's nothing we love more than having to haul our strollers out into the street to get around your trash bin. How about putting it at the end of your walkway next time, like the rest of the civilized world?

6. People who don't have accessible entrances

Hey, store owner. We want your coffee / your cute accessories / your cool furniture, we really do. But we don't want it badly enough to drag our strollers up your stupid, annoying steps. Get it together.

7. People who set off fireworks after 8:00 p.m. on stat holidays

Fuck you, people. We spend the entire duration of your pyromaniacal fun praying the POW POW POW doesn't wake our baby and throw off our sleep schedule.

8. People who wear strong perfume

Yes, you, old lady wearing Elizabeth Taylor's 'White Diamonds'. Thanks to you we have to hose our babies down because you hugged them and now they're making us gag.

9. People (Babies) who bite / hit / pinch / kick your kid

In our heads, we know that the biter / hitter / pincher / kicker in question is literally just a baby, but in our hearts, we still hate them a little bit.

10. People who don't give up their seat on public transit to pregnant women

Don't pretend you don't see that poor lady with her swollen belly, holding her lower back. Her pelvis probably feels like it's about to implode and her equilibrium is totally messed up due to the giant ball of human attached to her front side. But yeah, don't bother getting up.

HOW TO GET FIVE GODDAMN MINUTES TO YOURSELF

Everyone with a young child has been in this scenario before: you're unshowered and exhausted, in the middle of feeding your kid dinner (while simultaneously tackling endless loads of dishes and laundry), when your partner gets home and casually strolls right past you and into the bathroom. Seconds later, you hear the faint but distinct sound of video content coming out of an iPhone speaker. All you can think in that moment is, *"Is this motherfucker is taking a break? A BREAK? When they've been home for ten minutes, and I've been here grinding for the past fourteen hours?!"*

Oh, hell no.

If you're currently in the early part of the newborn phase and you're thinking, "Maybe *some* partners (let's be honest - men) are like that, but not my man. He is so helpful and attentive! If anything, he encourages me to take breaks!" We hope that continues for you, girl, we really do. From our experience, when a baby is in the super-sleepy / lazy newborn phase, the desire to escape for a hot minute doesn't really come into play. Once that baby becomes a bit louder and a bit more demanding, however, it seems that dads everywhere miraculously discover their underlying Irritable Bowel Syndrome.

It's time to expose their not-so-secret break-behaviour and take back our freedom (even if that freedom only comes in five-to-ten-minute increments). Here's how to beat them at their own clever game:

◊◊◊

1. Say you have to run to the store to get tampons: Men are afraid of tampons, and they hate buying them. They're never going to say, "Don't worry, babe, I'll just grab them for you on my lunch tomorrow." Use the tampon excuse to go to the drugstore, wander aimlessly through the aisles, and buy yourself a new lipstick.

2. Say you're going to go do the laundry: Men don't know what happens in the basement and they don't want to know. Bring your phone with you, toss in a load of towels, then sit on the stairs scrolling mindlessly for ten blissful minutes.

3. Take up a hobby that's as "serious" as his: "I have to go to yoga on Friday, because I really can't let the other yogis in my class down!" He doesn't know how yoga works. Go team!

4. Say you're going to have a bath with the kid(s): Fill the tub half-way, get yourself and the baby / babies undressed, hop in the bath, wash them down quickly, then yell, "HEY, BABE! THE KIDS ARE CLEAN; CAN YOU COME GET THEM?" Once they have been removed from the tub, say, "Can you shut the door, please?" Turn on the hot water, throw some Epsom salts up in there, and enjoy. If you're a planner, toss a bottle of wine and a wineglass in the cabinet beforehand.

5. Say you have to prepare *(insert something very complicated-sounding here)* for the baby: Go into the kitchen, pour yourself a cup of tea - or a little Bourbon on the rocks - and get into the groove. The baby DOES need to eat, after all. (P.S. This is why your grandma always kicked you out of the kitchen when you were little; it was never about the possibility of you burning yourself on the stove.)

6. Say you need to change the linens: Men have no idea what this actually entails, meaning they have no concept of how much time it takes to do it. Bring your phone with you, call a friend, write down some creative ideas, creep people on Facebook, watch TV in your room, WHATEVER! You just scored yourself half-an-hour of me-time.

7. Announce that YOU need to use the bathroom: Your tummy's not feeling great. Maybe mention your period, too. Whatever it takes. If you need a few minutes in a hurry, this will get you there.

8. Play the honesty card: On some level, every partner knows that we mamas are overworked and underappreciated, so if you need a breather, just get up and say, "I need five goddamn minutes to myself." Go lay in your bed in shavasana, take the dog for a walk around the block, or stand in the shower and let the hot water beat down on your sore shoulders. Don't forget to lock the door.

CHILDCARE DILEMMAS

Back when we were in the throes of solving our post-maternity-leave childcare probs, we were beyond stressed out. So many variables to account for, so many pros and cons to consider, SO MUCH PRESSURE.

Not only does this decision have the potential to make or break your career, but it also comes at a time when your kid is clingy AF. To make matters worse, the thought of leaving your child in the care of anyone other than you is often accompanied by both guilt and fear.

The good news is that young children are extremely adaptable. Give them a nanny and they're best friends after twenty minutes at the park. Hand them to the grandparents, they'll be playing gin rummy and shooting craps before you know it. Send them to daycare, and by week two, they'll have ten new friends and won't want you walking them all the way to the classroom door anymore, because they'll prefer to do it alone "like a big kid."

Our suggestion? Take a close look at your family's unique situation and make a childcare decision based on that. Don't base your decision on what your friends are doing or what the latest study on "future childhood success" has just revealed. Base this decision on your little crew and your collective happiness, and nothing more.

We personally put a lot of thought (and research) into making the grand childcare decision for our families. Since the whole ordeal was a giant pain in the ass for us, we figured we'd save you the trouble and delve into all the options on your behalf. You've got enough shit to do these days, right?

CHILDCARE OPTION	PROS	CONS
STAY-AT-HOME MOM/DAD	You get to be home for all the BIG moments.	You're stuck at home through all the day-to-day crap.
	No scrambling for childcare if your kid gets sick.	If your kid gets sick, you're probably next.
	Your kid won't be exposed to all the germs and grossness of a daycare facility.	Your kid's immune system won't get the early boost from all the germs and grossness of a daycare facility.
	You get to pick when/ with whom your kid socializes.	You are solely responsible for socializing your kid, meaning you too will have to socialize (and the moms at the park may make you want to claw out your left eye).
	You don't have to go to work.	You risk setting yourself back in your career trajectory.
	Play dates involve your baby socializing and YOU socializing, which is awesome if you've got some bad-ass mom friends. Did somebody say afternoon sangria?	You may begin to feel like your kid's personal assistant.
	When you're having a shit day, you can literally stay in your pyjamas for as long as you damn well please.	You may end up spending more time in your pyjamas than you're comfortable with.
WORK-FROM HOME MOM/DAD	You get to be home for all the BIG moments.	You're stuck at home, trying to work during unpredictable nap windows.
	You get more of a work/life balance.	You'll feel like it's more of a work/life juggling act / freak show.
	You'll make your own schedule.	You'll have to make that schedule around your kid's schedule.

CHILDCARE OPTION	PROS	CONS
	You'll surprise yourself with what you can accomplish in short, sporadic windows of time.	Any "downtime" you thought you'd have will be spent working.
DAYCARE	Your kid will be interacting and socializing with other kids all day.	Your kid will bring ALL OF THE GERMS home.
	You will be able to go back to work.	It's so expensive that you'll likely just be handing your pay-cheque over to the daycare centre.
	You won't be stuck at home, dealing with the day-to-day crap.	You'll probably miss some of the BIG moments.
	You'll drink in every minute you spend with your little one. (Absence makes the heart grow fonder!)	You'll never feel like you've had enough time with your little one.
	Your kid will become more adaptable.	Adjusting to a slightly more uncomfortable environment may result in some temporary behavioural pushback.
	Free. Time.	Drop-offs may be emotional torture.
NANNY	Freedom to work from home or out of the house, knowing your kid can stick to his regular routine while you do it.	You'll have to deal with the distraction of having your kid all over you if you're home.
	Extra set of hands to help with childcare and other household duties.	The price tag that comes with such a luxury.
	The ability to choose the perfect person to help out on the home front.	The pressure and time commitment that comes with choosing the perfect person to help out on the home front.

CHILDCARE OPTION	PROS	CONS
	The possibility of a wonderful, long-lasting relationship with the person you hire.	The possibility of a disastrous, short-lived relationship with the person you hire.
	Flexible work-hours.	The price tag that comes with the luxury of flexible work-hours.
	Your house. Your Rules.	Your empty bank account.
GRANDPARENT OR OTHER FAMILY MEMBER	Probably free!	Possibly unreliable.
	Your kid gets to form a close bond with the designated family member.	The designated family member will likely spoil the shit out of your kid.
	Your kid gets someone's undivided love and attention all day (plus, there's always the park or library drop-in they can attend to make baby friends).	Your kid probably won't get as many opportunities to socialize with kids their age as they would at a daycare.
	If you're lucky, this caregiver will also cook (common amongst the grands).	You'll have to relinquish your control-freak health-food ways and just be glad you're not the one doing all the cooking anymore.

DRESSING LIKE A REBEL MAMA

Whether we like it or not, having a baby changes the way we dress, but that doesn't have to be a bad thing. After all, jeans and a t-shirt has always been the quintessential cool-girl uniform, and casual, laid-back style will always be en vogue.

Once your post-baby weight loss begins to plateau, it may be time to treat yourself to a few wardrobe essentials to get you through the next little while without muffin-topping out of your pre-baby jeans or drowning in your maternity leggings.

WARNING: the fitting room may be a traumatic space for you right now. Wall-to-wall mirrors revealing every new fold, bulge, and stretch mark may feel like the stuff of postpartum nightmares, but trust us when we tell you that buying just a few key pieces that fit and flatter will change your life for months to come.

Pro Tips:

- Try to procure your new "micro wardrobe" during sale time. You don't want to break the bank in case your body changes shape yet again in the near future (ours did three or four times before settling in for good). Hold out until June/July for spring-summer sales, and December/January for fall-winter sales.

- Go on your hunt in the morning during the week. The stores will be quiet, and you can nab a sales associate to help you. Ask them to grab different sizes and help you navigate the styles they carry. You know you've picked the right person if they tell you that something's not flattering and then bring you something better to try.

- Hit up Pinterest and Instagram for inspiration. We take our cues from the queens of effortless, laid-back style: Caroline de Maigret, Jane Birkin, Kate Moss, and Pernille Teisbaek.

- Do not buy anything that can't be easily cleaned at home. There will be a time and place again for dry-clean only, but it's not right now.

- Before you go shopping, go through your current wardrobe and toss anything that has no business being there. You know the stuff we're talking about: the party top from 2009, the sweat pants from college, and the jeans you haven't fit into for over five years. Take a page from Marie Kondo: If it brings you no joy, it needs to go. Make room for stuff that makes you feel good.

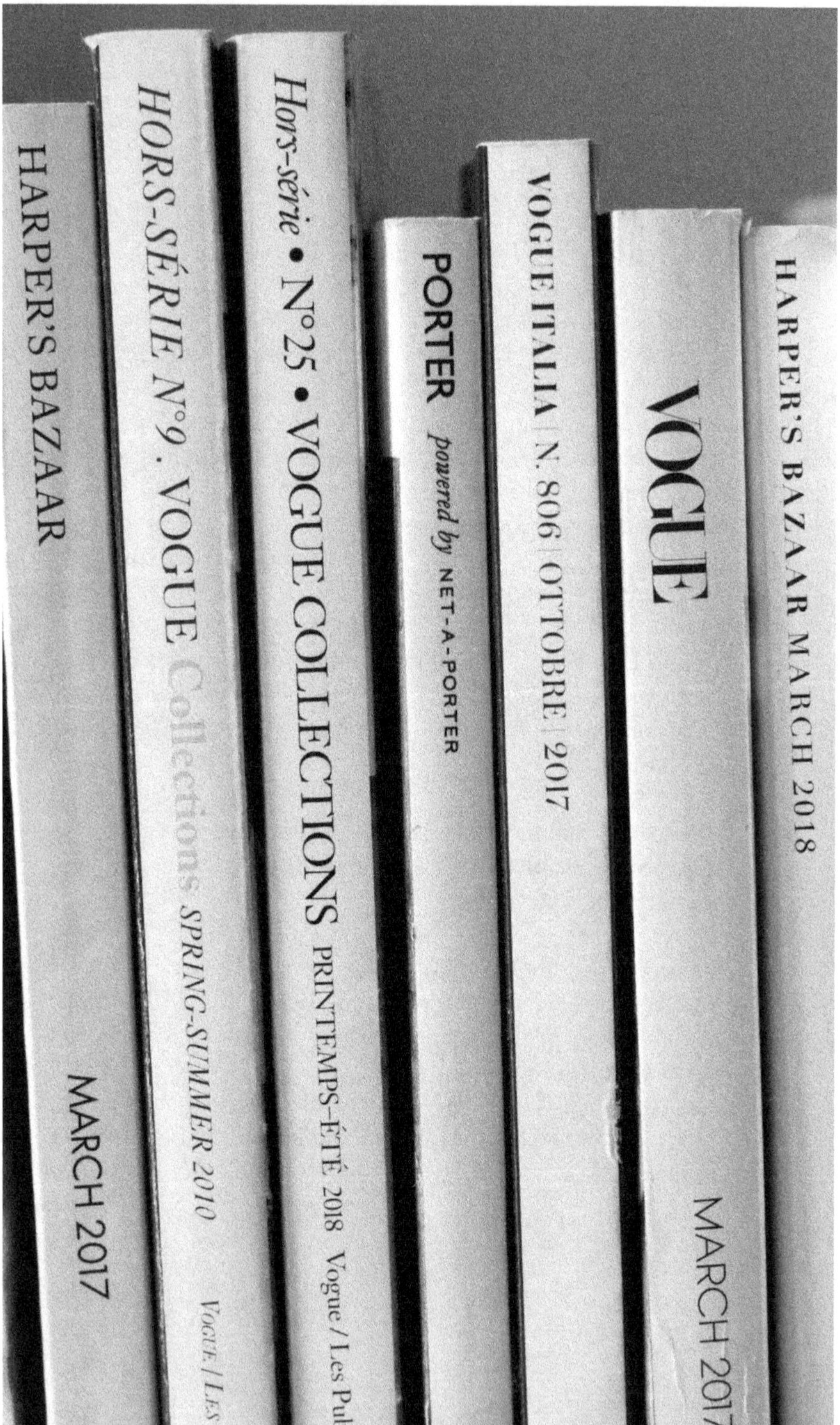
HARPER'S BAZAAR
MARCH 2017
HORS-SÉRIE N°9. VOGUE Collections SPRING-SUMMER 2010
VOGUE / LES P
Hors-série • N°25 • VOGUE COLLECTIONS PRINTEMPS-ÉTÉ 2018
Vogue / Les Publi
PORTER powered by NET-A-PORTER
VOGUE ITALIA | N. 806 | OTTOBRE | 2017
VOGUE
MARCH 2017
HARPER'S BAZAAR MARCH 2018

Now for the fun part: what to buy. There are a few basics that every Rebel Mama will benefit from adding to her wardrobe.

1. Jeans (one or two pairs)

There's something about zipping up a good pair of jeans that makes you feel like a functioning member of society. Look for mid-to-high-rise styles in a solid wash (the darker the wash, the more forgiving the jeans). You want a pair with some stretch, but not so much stretch that they feel like leggings (denim that's too soft will lose its shape quickly). Keep in mind that tailoring denim is key. Your sales associate should be able to help you decide whether it needs a little cinch at the waist or a taper or hem at the ankle. You know you've found the right pair when you feel five-pounds lighter in them than you felt when you walked into the store.

2. Basic Tees (about five of them)

No writing, no bells or whistles. You need a simple, well-fitted tee that works well either un-tucked or half-tucked. In order to achieve the perfect half-tuck, grab the bottom of the tee, twist it a bit to one side and tuck in ONLY the part that you're holding. This creates subtle ruching that immediately flatters your midsection and elongates your legs.

Once you find this tee, buy multiples. Black, white, beige, grey, navy, striped, and done.

3. Sneakers

Ever since "athleisure wear" became a trend, you can pretty much get a cool pair of kicks anywhere. High end, low end, basic, bedazzled. There truly is something for everyone.

Note: If it all seems too overwhelming, classic white Converse will never fail you.

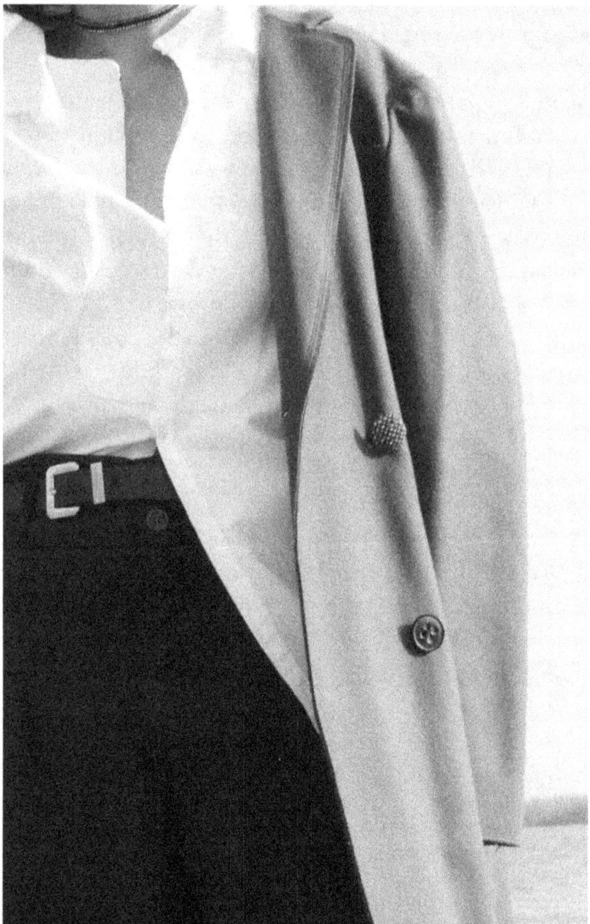

4. Actual Shoes (that aren't sneakers)

If you live in a climate that has multiple seasons, take advantage of fall dressing and go get a gorgeous new shoe or boot with a medium heel, that is comfortable to walk in (meaning not a stiletto, for most of us), to wear during the day. You should be so in love with these that you'd pick them over your sneakers any day, because they make you feel like a mega babe.

Also, take your existing shoes that look a little beat up to a cobbler for a face-lift. You'd be surprised at how shiny and new they'll look and feel afterwards. Never underestimate the value of fresh-looking footwear.

5. A Leather Jacket

Go on a hunt for an awesome leather jacket (our go-to is a classic black biker-style). If you break the bank on one thing, this should be it. A good leather jacket should be timeless. It can be fitted or slightly oversized - both are cool in their own way. You'll know you've found the right jacket when you feel like a rock star in it. It should be something you'd be comfortable throwing on with jeans and a tee or over a little black dress.

6. A Structured Blazer

This is another classic item that easily transforms your go-to jeans and tees. Wear to a dinner party with fun costume jewelry or out for lunch with your sneakers and a baseball hat. Generally speaking, if it hits you halfway down your butt, it will be a flattering length. Buy this wardrobe essential from a store with actual sales people, who genuinely know what they're doing, and it will be well worth the investment.

Go with whatever size fits your shoulders and then let a tailor do the rest. Tailors are as close as we regular people get to made-to-measure, custom clothing. Your goal here is to create long, vertical lines, which will make you look taller and slimmer. A well-tailored blazer can even make your waistline appear smaller.
Can we get a hallelujah?

7. A Pair of Cool Shades

Sunglasses are a mom's best friend. They cover tired eyes better than any bb cream or under-eye concealer on the market. They are also a totally justifiable treat due to their cost-per-wear value (take the cost and divide it by the amount of times you think you'll wear it. Apply this calculation to all the pieces suggested above to pull off this shopping spree guilt-free).

8. Accessories

When you're working with a capsule wardrobe, your accessories make the difference between a coffee-with-a-girlfriend outfit and a dinner-with-your-man outfit. Let's say you decide to wear your favourite jeans and a tee with your leather jacket on top to your coffee date. All you need to do to bring this outfit from day to night is add a statement earring, a bold lip colour, some sexy stilettos, et voilà!

◊◊◊

Simplifying your wardrobe (especially for a new mom) can and should be looked at as an act of self-love. In addition to feeling great, you're also giving yourself the gift of having to make one less decision in a day. Steve Jobs wore the same thing every day. So does Mark Zuckerberg. Why is that? Because they have more important shit to think about every day, and so do you.

When you're laying the foundation upon which to build your newly simplified wardrobe, take care to select key pieces that reflect the woman you are (with a dash of the woman you wish to be).

Invest in quality. Look semi-groomed (that means slicking back your unwashed hair into a sleek ponytail), feel confident, be your beautiful self, and feel like the bad-ass mama you are.

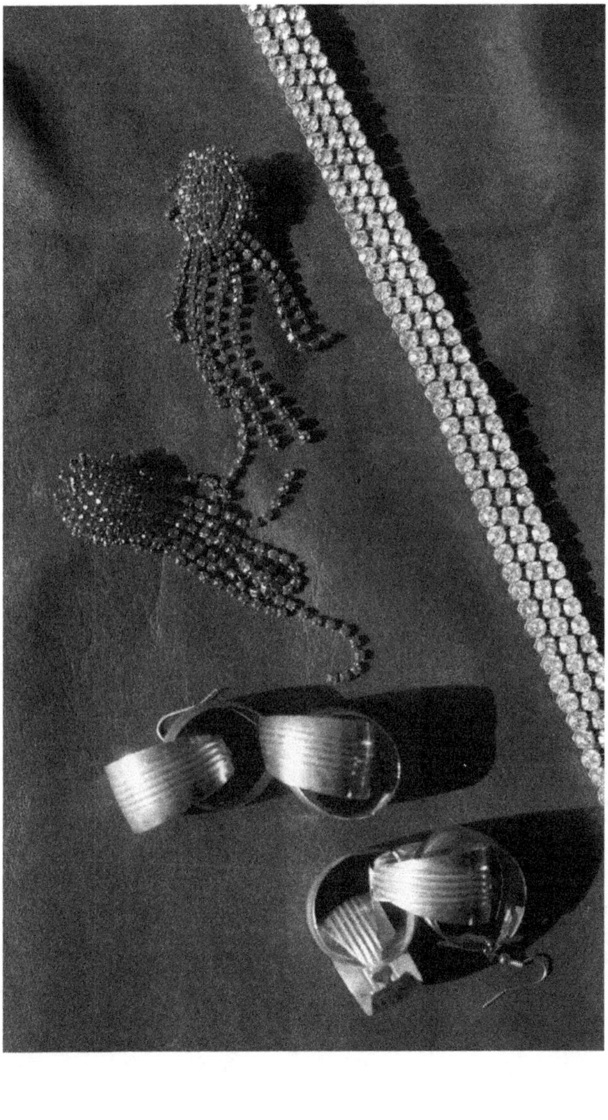

Part 4
ON TODDLERS

"We spend the first twelve months of our children's lives teaching them to walk and talk, and the next twelve telling them to sit down and shut up."

– Phyllis Diller

UNSOLICITED
RAPID-FIRE ADVICE

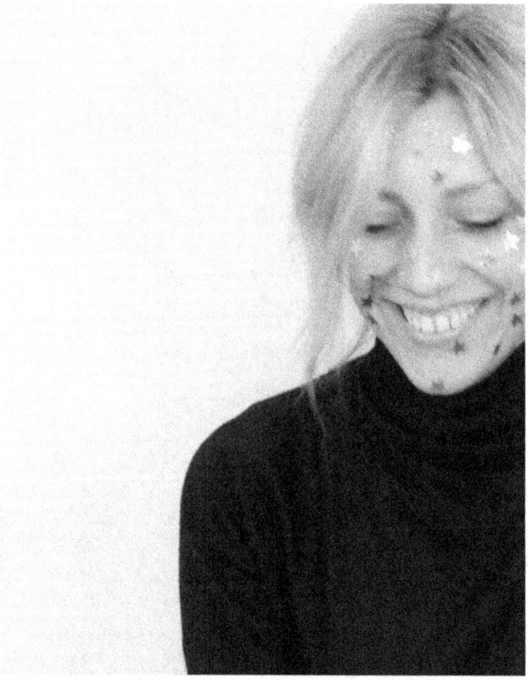

◊ Always have mini M&Ms on hand for unforeseen bribery opportunities.

◊ Add a pinch of cayenne pepper to your morning coffee for an added boost of energy without having to resort to cocaine.

◊ Google image "Kids Rotten Teeth" to really drive home the point about brushing every day. Much more powerful than some sing-a-long song.

◊ Stick your kid in a large empty box, fill it with crayons/markers/stickers, call it a "craft fort", then enjoy twenty minutes of precious alone time.

◊ Add a shot of Irish Cream to your coffee on days where you *just can't* and it's only 8:00 a.m.

◊ So over the soother in your kid's mouth? Cut a slit in it. No suction = no fun.

◊ Trick your kids into napping by telling them they are only allowed to sleep for ONE HOUR. They will fight you and demand two hours, at which point you can say, "OK, FINE! Have it your way."

◊ Purée frozen bananas alone or with cocoa, peanut butter, or Bailey's (oops, we meant *berries*) and BAM! Homemade ice-cream.

◊ Make your kid a makeup bag of brushes, mirrors, etc, of their own so they can leave your Sephora shit alone while you're getting ready.

◊ Google "overnight oats." Your only breakfast duty the next day will be a fresh pot of coffee.

◊ Fill up empty soap dispensers with bubble bath and water for a seriously fun bath-time game. Sit back and watch the magic unfold, preferably with a glass of wine in hand.

◊ Send them for a sleepover at Grandma's for no reason. They'll get spoiled rotten, you'll sleep in until 8:00 a.m., and you'll wake to a clean and quiet house.

◊ Use puppy-training sheets to put under your almost-fully-potty-trained toddler's fitted sheets so the mattress doesn't get destroyed.

◊ Use an empty plastic egg carton for paints and water. Clean up: the lazy kind.

◊ Use Band-Aids as temporary outlet covers when travelling.

YOUR DRUNK FRIEND FROM COLLEGE 2.0

There's something that parents of young children rarely like to admit, much less discuss, and it's the fact that toddlers are fucking crazy.

Being the mom of a toddler means dealing with an unpredictable, spatially unaware, politically incorrect little human day in and day out.

Nobody ever fully warned us about just how insane this phase would be. Sure, they mentioned that "they're a handful" and told us to "wait 'til the Terrible Twos," but that's all abstract bullshit. What we really needed was something that we could genuinely relate to, an easy comparison to help prepare us for life avec toddler. It's too late for us now, since we're already residents of Toddlerville, but we finally came up with the perfect analogy that we hope will help you understand what's coming your way.

Remember that really drunk friend you had in college? The one that you somehow developed a soft spot for? The one who incessantly begged you to go to McDonald's with him after the party? The one you always ended up taking home with you because you thought he would definitely manage to kill himself at some point between the front door and his bed?

Well, that friend is back. Except this time, he's only two feet tall. Yep, your toddler is just a tiny drunk person, and it's your job to keep him fed, watered, and rested. Bonus points if you can manage to get him to not act like a wild animal in public.

When he gets belligerent and starts demanding that he eat something *immediately,* the nearest fast-food joint won't cut it. Instead, you'll have to carefully prepare a fully organic meal for him, and if he doesn't like what you've made, he's going to nonchalantly throw that shit on the floor, right in front of you.

God help you if you need to leave the house with him in tow. Prepare yourself for the biggest production of life. It won't matter how many times you tell him he's putting his boots on the wrong feet, he'll just pretend he can't hear you.

If/when you do make it out of the house, you'd better watch him like a fucking hawk. His lack of balance means he'll be knocking over displays left, right, and centre. He'll incessantly beg you to buy him a bag of Goldfish crackers and insist on opening a juice box while you're still roaming the aisles. Don't be surprised if he tries to steal a chocolate bar in the checkout line; this dude cannot be trusted.

He'll laugh at the most inappropriate times, randomly refuse to wear pants, and if he decides to go to the washroom, there WILL be pee on the floor for you to clean up afterwards.

Once he's done destroying your powder room, he'll come out ready to chat, and you better believe he's going to tell you the same damn story over and over and over again until it's finally time to try to coerce him into going to bed. Here's how that's going to go down: Step 1: Catch him, hold him down, and force him to brush his teeth. Step 2: Try to get him into his pyjamas as he thrashes all over the place and somehow turns his limbs into Jell-O, making the whole process impossible. Step 3: Ignore all his talk of "not being tired"- it's a hoax. Once he gets upstairs, he likely won't even be able to get both feet up on the bed before passing out completely.

Once he's been sleeping for a few hours and you finally decide to break out the "good" wine and cuddle up with your partner, he'll reveal himself to be the worst third wheel of all time. Like clockwork, the minute you get cozy on the couch, you'll hear, "I'm thirsty! Water!! Juice!! Thiiiiirrrrssttttyyyy!!!" and up you'll go to make sure he's hydrated, to remind him that it's "night-night time," and to tell him not to bug you again until morning (HAHA).

Good luck!

BABY TALK
(AND THE ART OF NOT USING IT)

We'd like to preface this by saying that there is one exception to the "no baby talk" rule, and that's when you're dealing with an actual baby (under the age of one). For these super tiny beings, baby talk helps them understand rhythm of speech, helps you to bond with them, blah, blah, blah. But once they're older than one, you're done.

Nothing grates our nerves more than listening to a grown-ass woman saying things like, "Are you a sicky bear? Is your widdle bum bum ouchy? Does my peanut-butter-jelly-cup need to go caca?"

Nope.

If your kid's at an age of pseudo talking (somewhere between one and two-years-old) and can muster up a simple yet clear enough sentence (read: "Mama. I dunnwanna nap.") then take this as your OFFICIAL cue to drop the game and introduce them to the art of (a) conversation, and (b) conveying actual information.

The words we choose are important, and a child is never too young to know them and use them properly. Sometimes we can get in the habit of over-simplifying things for the little ones, without realizing that babies and toddlers are way smarter than we give them credit for.

Children have the capacity to understand bigger and better words. Flower, dog, and bird are fine for the first round, but who wants to keep that conversation going for long? New words are easy to find if you just open your eyes. *Equipment. Asphalt. Eucalyptus. Hand rail. Apricot. Lavender.* See? Much better.

Descriptive words are awesome, because you can legitimately go on and on while your kid just soaks it up like a sponge. It's not just a blue truck that goes "beep beep" (save that for hungover parenting); it's a *recycling truck* that *recycles packaging* like *plastic, paper, and cardboard,* to help us *keep the planet healthy and green.* Look at all those awesome words!

Choosing words carefully and speaking clearly (and politely) will eventually rub off on your little one. The more natural and confident your kid gets with composing a strong sentence, the more respect they'll gain at school, in the sandbox, and a couple of decades down the line, at the killer dinner party that you won't be invited to.

Finally, listening is also a huge part of proper communication. Teach your new conversationalist to listen and not interrupt, and extend the same courtesy to them. Leading by example is the most effective parenting tactic around.

WHO'S THE BOSS?

If you've got kids, then the answer is you. YOU are the fucking boss.

Mamas, we can't afford to lose the never-ending power struggle. We can't end up in a place where we're literally asking our children if they'd like to eat their greens, *as if they have the ability to make a well-informed decision on the matter.*

When did dessert become a given, rather than a treat or a privilege? Are we seriously letting our tiny and completely irrational spawns make decisions for themselves that could result in diabetes, obesity, and malnutrition? We need to cut that shit out, and fast. When we consult our kids about basic care-giving matters like what to eat or when to go to bed, they don't feel taken care of. They freak out and take on the alpha role in the relationship, and disaster ensues.

There has been a massive shift in parenting over the last few decades. As Millennials (cue eye rolls from everyone else), we are the generation of participation ribbons. Even though we're educated AF and have made some incredible contributions, a lot of us were never fully able to break away from the teat. Our parents help us with down payments on our houses, they throw us some cash if our Visa bill gets out of control, and they occasionally show up at our condos with groceries or home-cooked meals. We have been *the kid* our whole lives, even after we became *adults.* Is it that surprising that, as parents, we are totally uncomfortable being the boss?

We want everyone to get along. We want our kids to like us, and we want them to feel like we genuinely respect their opinions. We want our homes to be democracies, not dictatorships. But we're being stupid and short-sighted. What we're doing with our would-you-like-to-have-a-bath-tonights and our are-you-ready-to-go-to-bed-yets is creating a generation of sleep-deprived, sugar-infused people who think that the world revolves around them, and who truly believe that even their most ridiculous desires deserve attention and *fulfillment.* Terrifying.

Now that we know this is a problem, what can we do to stop it?

For starters, we can stop with the goddamn questions. Some things are non-negotiable, and we don't want our kids thinking otherwise. It's time to make a conscious effort to change the rhetoric we use in our homes. For example, instead of saying, "Can you help Mama clean up this mess you made, please?" say, "Before we can play another game, you need to help clean up." Simple, direct, *and not a fucking question.*

The same goes for anything related to other non-negotiables, namely food and sleep. Paying close attention to word choices is super helpful in reducing occurrences of power confusion. For example, instead of asking your kids if they *"want"* to eat their lunch, and if they could *"please have a bite of this sandwich for mommy,"* your priority should be making sure your kids don't think that mealtime is optional, or that they're doing you any favours by eating.

We need them to know who's in charge, and the best way we can do that is to make it very clear that, until they can make rational decisions for themselves, everything pertaining to their health and well-being is strictly under parental jurisdiction. Anything else is fair game. For example, here are some questions you could gladly ask your kids (and happily acquiesce to their responses):

- What would you like to wear today?
- Which park should we go to?
- What books do you want to read this afternoon?
- Would you prefer broccoli or peas? (this one's a trick question - either way, they're eating greens)
- Should we colour? Or do stickers?

Autonomy can still be taught without completely disrupting the parent / child paradigm. Maybe some of you are sitting there thinking, *Wow, mean-mommy much?* But the fact remains that in order for kids to flourish intellectually, emotionally, and creatively, they need to know that there is a responsible adult in their corner who has their absolute best interests in mind. So, let us ask you this one more time: In your household, **WHO'S THE BOSS?**

THE KIDS ARE ALRIGHT.

iCHOOSE SANITY: A (REALISTIC) GUIDE TO SCREEN TIME

We keep a few "rules" in our back pockets regarding screen time, but for the most part, we're done feeling guilty about exactly how many minutes our kids clock per day. Ain't nobody got time for that.

If you're looking for a magic formula, here it is: there is no magic formula. Do what you have to do to get shit done, even if it means putting the curated toys away for a little modern animation. When the energy in the house starts to get stale, power down and head outdoors or bust out the books and crafts. Trust your gut on this one, Mama. And if it makes you feel less shitty, throw on something "educational" and call it a day.

Here are some rules that we mostly (sometimes) adhere to:

- If they're going to watch TV, they are going to watch good TV. Not all children's programming is unbearable, and *Sesame Street* is still as rad as it was in 1987. Bonus Tip: Keep the volume low to allow them to lose interest; your ears will thank you.

- When eating out, screens are a no-go. We respect and value the restaurant industry way too much to take the whole experience away from the child. With practice and patience, they will learn to endure it, enjoy it, and even embrace basic social human interaction. Note: obviously, in extreme meltdown situations, -the screen has been drawn.

- When they do steal your phone (and they will), sell them on the coolest parts, i.e. NOT the Internet. Get them into family photos and Google Map journeys rather than mindless streams. Take it up a notch and teach your spawn to take majestic photos of you.

- Keep a safe distance. A good rule of thumb is to make a fist with the child's hand under their chin. The distance between their face and their elbow is as close as the screen should be.

- Don't use screens in the dark; it's not good for their little eyeballs.

- Set time limits. Unless it's an emergency, it's going into shut down mode after half an hour and kiddo is free to figure out what else they'd like to do with their infinite amounts of free time. If the grab-n-go doesn't go over well, blame dying batteries.

- Find educational and engaging games online and get your kid learning early. It will make you feel like a genius mom when your babe knows his ABCs before the other sandbox tenants. Bonus: This will save your ass on flights.

At the end of the day, it comes down to balance. If your child spends tons of time outside, is well socialized, and exposed to a plethora of activities that don't include screens, an episode (or three) of *Thomas the Train* won't kill anyone, especially when you're on toenail-cutting duty.

We are all trying to live alongside technology and not be ruled by it, so here's hoping we can disconnect from time to time and enjoy the simple pleasures of life without going into withdrawal. Is there anything on the Internet that can truly beat a picnic in the park? (If you answered porn or online shopping, you need to throw your phone in a lake immediately.)

Children learn from watching us, so as long as we have healthy digital habits, they will too. As long as we don't have our phones strapped to our foreheads 24/7 and can carry on a decent conversation, the kids will be alright.

POTTY TRAINING: DON'T BOTHER

Once you're on a mission to potty train (probably because some 18-month-old at Gymboree was touting boxer briefs last week, prompting you to think your 2-year-old has fallen behind developmentally - she hasn't), chances are you will fall into the consumerist trap that is "The Potty-Training Essentials."

The only true Potty-Training Essentials are (1) patience (because this process will involve someone inevitably peeing on your sofa and/or rug); (2) self-restraint (try not to lose your shit as you scrape someone else's shit out of a pair of skivvies); and (3) common sense (to snap you out of wanting to buy into 800 gimmicks - just grab a training seat that goes onto the existing toilet, a bunch of extremely small underwear, and bribes. Always bribes).

The only time a toddler is going to shit in a toilet is whenever she goddamn pleases.

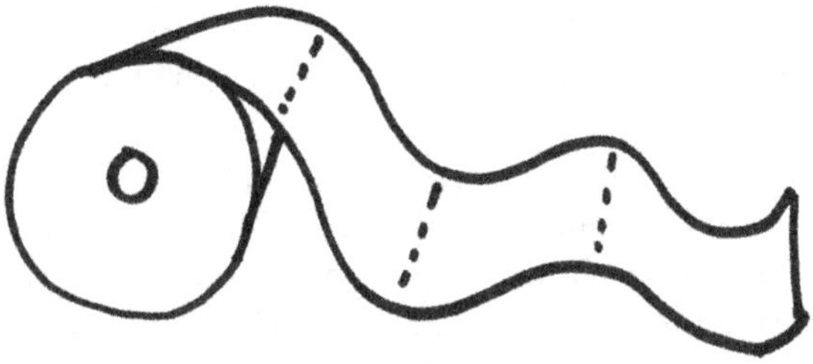

AVOIDING THE OVER-GIFTING EPIDEMIC

We don't know about you, but we can't focus on a damn thing if our homes aren't in perpetual *Vogue Living* status. Beyond the fact that it doesn't look or feel good, hoarding loads of useless junk is not good for anyone's soul, especially not a child's.

Naturally, when our friends and family kept showing up bearing noisy, plastic, light-up toys that only added clutter to our spaces (that we work so hard to keep uncluttered), we had to figure out a way to put a stop to it.

First and foremost, your child does not actually need (or want, for that matter) all those toys. Kids were also around hundreds of years ago, and they developed just fine without Tickle-Me-Elmo (sorry, bro).

It's also likely that your child already owns thirteen variations of whatever new Tonka truck he just received, and because he's got the attention span of a small rodent, he will play with this novelty item for a few days (a week at most) and then it will be forgotten, discarded, and left to die a slow death under a pile of snow in the backyard. Remind the gift-givers of this.

If you're like us, you already work really damn hard to simplify your kid's childhood in an era of over-consumption and instant gratification. Let would-be gift-givers know that you'd rather nurture your child's curiosity by exposing them to the world around them (a.k.a. the outdoors), and that you're trying to teach your kid that people and experiences matter more than "things."

We haven't even touched on the incredible amount of waste that is destroying our environment. We are ALL responsible for our consumption, and that applies to children's toys too.

That's why we're imploring you to ask your village to get creative about birthdays / holidays / showers / etc. Be the leader and encourage others to live by your example. You, your home, your recycling bin, your local playground, and your child will all be better for it.

Some ideas:

- Splurging on a new baby is fine - everyone is allowed to purchase one incredibly adorable outfit or toy that is begging to be Instagrammed. Just not upon every damn visit. Make that clear.

- If they're fixated with buying your babe a toy, suggest getting something they can both get involved in. A ball, a paint set, Play-Doh, puzzles, Lego - all of those things are better together.

- Remind them that kids love ridiculously simple things. If they come over with a bag of balloons, they're guaranteed a positive reaction.

- Books, books, and more books. In the age of TV, iPads, and Smartphones, your kid will need to balance out all of that screen time. Books never get old. They are loved, passed down, and used over and over until the pages are worn.

- The gift of music has the ability to transcend time and speak in a language everyone can understand. It teaches, it unifies, it evokes feelings, and it triggers the imagination. Whether it's an instrument, records, or even a Spotify subscription, music is life. Encourage gift-givers to keep that in mind.

- Rally your crew into doing something with your kid. Taking the bus across the city to bite into the best pizza slice in town can be an adventure of epic proportions.

- A stroll through a new park or playground in a different neighbourhood makes a glorious gift. Extra points if they get down and dirty exploring bugs with your mini-scientist.

- Ask them to babysit and go wherever they please for a few hours. Not only will this buy you some much-needed alone time, but they also get to choose their own adventure and learn something new about their city in the process.

- If they're aching to add some new clothes to the never-ending pile in your kid's dresser, remind them to check in with you first, as you may be in the market for a new raincoat as opposed to the newest baby Air Jordans.

- Are monster trucks your child's latest obsession? Look into when the monster-truck show is coming to town and make it a family trip. Kiddo into dinosaur bones? The museum's got 'em and they are gigantic and amazing. Little sports fan on your hands? Suggest a blissfully boring baseball game and pack in some quality time in the sun.

- Most importantly, drive this concept home: **Experiences over toys. Memories over stuff.**

And if Grandma is still hell bent on spending some money, advise her to drive to the local liquor store and snag you ladies some Pinot Noir.

THE THREENAGER

We hate to be the bearers of bad news, but just because you survived the "terrible twos" does not put you in the clear. In fact, you're on the cusp of a whole new and (believe it or not) scarier phase of toddlerhood.

Defiance. Rebellion. Incessant whining. Taunting. Scheming. Little white lies. Random acts of violence. Dramatic outbursts. Mood swings. And our personal favourite: selective hearing.

Meet "THE THREENAGER".

When did they become so smart? When did they become so emotionally unstable? WHEN THE HELL DID THEY LEARN TO ROLL THEIR DAMN EYES? These little tyrants have no right to be cranky assholes after a two-hour nap, while being served an array of fruit, and choosing a Netflix show. We're running a Five Star Hotel over here.

Here are some things that have recently come out of the mouths of our threenagers:

- I'm annoying. You're annoying.
- It's not interesting, this food.
- Okay, you need to relax, babe.
- I'm cutting you off.
- I want to go outside, but I don't want to get dirty.
- It's not an option.
- I'm tired. Because my penis is tired.
- You're a disaster.
- I'm gonna go naked. With my nipples.
- I cannnnn't. I just can't.
- I don't like rainbows.
- I have water. You have wine.
- THAT'S ALL I WILL SAY.
- I'm holding my penissssss.
- I have a plan. You have to listen to my plan.
- This park is too messy for me.
- I'm mad. I am NOT happy.

- Don't look at me!!
- I'm not gonna stay in bed. I'm telling you.
- I'm gonna kick you. You're bad, Mama.
- I'm gonna hold your hand, so you can focus.
- Can you just snuggle me today?
- I don't want to talk. It's a bad mood.
- Nobody touch me.
- I love you.

What can you do when you're stuck on the emotional roller-coaster that is the threenager (besides drowning in some kind of digestif and smoking your medicine dry)? Try to remember that it will end one day, and although you'll be relieved when they've eased up on driving you insane, you'll ironically miss it too (at least that's what we tell ourselves, so we don't constantly fly off the handle and end up with even more forehead wrinkles).

ADDITIONAL NOTES AND SURVIVAL TACTICS

Encourage your threenager to navigate all the crazy feels they're feeling, and teach them some coping mechanisms like basic breathing exercises. Sometimes when you're mad, taking a big, deep inhale followed by a really long exhale can make a huge difference. It will also buy you some silence.

Help them identify their feelings and understand their emotions a bit better. Say things like "I bet when that kid didn't want to play with you, it really made you feel sad, and maybe even a little embarrassed." Follow it up with "It's okay to feel that way. People feel that way all the time, including Mama! Now, go find a different game to play."

Next time shit starts going south, ask them to go sit on the stairs until they are ready to use their words to calmly tell you what's wrong. This reframes a time out in a way that allows you both to get the fuck away from each other for long enough to collect your thoughts and not make a bad situation worse.

If your kid is having an epic meltdown because you served their popcorn the wrong way, coolly explain (while trying really hard not to mock) how ridiculous that is, and move the hell on. Don't let them rope you into a twenty-minute whine fest about fucking popcorn. WALK AWAY, sister, walk away.

Make the decision not to take anything your threenager says or does personally and take every encounter with a grain of salt. Also, feel free to laugh about the whole situation (not in front of him, of course), because if you can't see the humour in your kid acting like a total jackass or saying things that are blatantly inappropriate, you're not going to survive this gig.

hahahahaha
(pass the bourbon)

HOW TO NOT LOSE YOUR SHIT ON THE DAILY

All moms lose their shit. Some moms may look like they have it all together, but trust us, they don't. They just have better ways of hiding it.

Below are some examples of the types of things that we tell ourselves when we need to haul ourselves out of the abyss. Feel free to borrow them whenever you feel the mom-crazy coming on. And remember: when in doubt, just calm the fuck down.

Scenario One

*You're mindlessly scrolling through the news on your phone and there it is: an article about a toddler who died (probably while their mom was scrolling through the news on her phone *insert mom guilt*). Panic sets in.*

Stop. Remember: tragedies are not the norm. Yes, they do happen. And yes, it's heartbreaking and awful when they do, but they really are rare. Pay attention to the world around you, but don't let yourself live in a place of fear. Everything is fine. We promise.

Scenario Two

It's been one of those days. Nothing is going right. The house looks like a bomb has been detonated in it, and all you want to do is teleport into the future to a time where the kids are self-sufficient and you can actually hear your own thoughts.

Stop. Remember: the days are long but the years are short. It's the most annoyingly true parenting cliché of all time. Whenever you feel like you want to press fast forward to your retirement plan, remind yourself of this mantra. Time feels like it's moving at a glacial pace sometimes (especially when your toddler starts the "incessant whining" phase), but it does fly by, and these childhood years make up a tiny percentage of your kid's life. Try to just breathe and take it all in. Try to remember all the little details - you'll be looking for them in your memory bank in the not-so-distant future.

Scenario Three

Your ever-confrontational spawn has you totally doubting your parenting abilities. In the span of one afternoon, you've lost your temper, you've yelled, you've thrown toys in the trash, and you've administered more time-outs than you'd like to admit. You wonder when this shit is going to get easier.

Stop. Remember: it's never going to get easier, but you're getting better every day. Every day you understand the need for patience more deeply. You muster more cojones to stick to your guns and set fair boundaries for your kids. You get more confident in your ability to make decisions on their behalf. Switch your goal from matronly perfection to constant improvement, and celebrate all the small wins. They're proof that you're moving in the right direction.

Scenario Four

Maybe you've put a career on hold to stay home with your kids. Maybe you've fallen into a bit of a slump, and you're feeling like you may never get your groove back. Either way, one day, when you're sitting in your living room, bored out of your tree as the Mickey Mouse Clubhouse theme song mocks you in the background, a "What have I done with my life?" freak-out ensues.

Stop. Remember: you've got time. Not to totally contradict point #2, but in the grand scheme of things, life is not even close to over yet, and there are opportunities to try new things every single day. Always remember that you're never too young or too old to change your mind and live life in a new way. If you want to try something - try it. Better an 'oops' than a 'what if'.

Part 5
ON SIBLINGS

"When my kids become wild and unruly, I use a nice, safe playpen. When they're finished, I climb out."

– Erma Bombeck

UNSOLICITED
RAPID-FIRE ADVICE

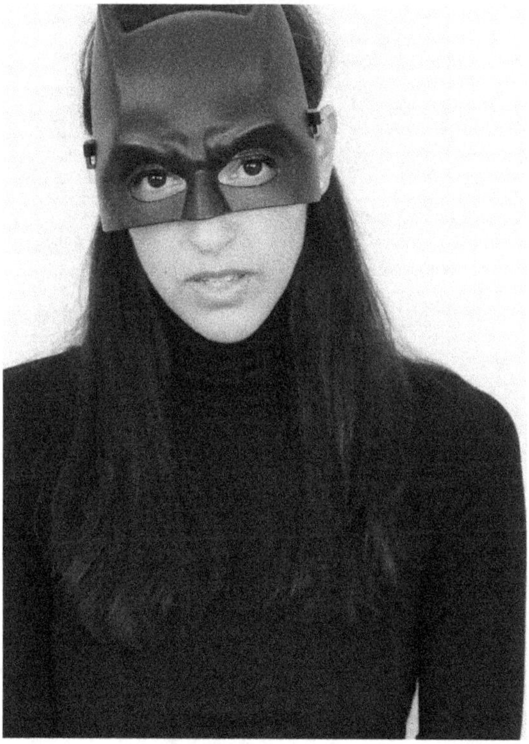

◊ Hype up the big-sibling thing, but not so much that your first-born thinks they have to be an adult now. Reminders that they'll always be your baby, even if they're the oldest, will be a huge source of comfort to them.

◊ Get over the guilt of not being as attentive with the second as you were with the first. It's a different game now. Different rules apply.

◊ The first few weeks/months with two is a shit show. Survival is the name of the game. Do whatever you need to do to get through the day and don't beat yourself up over ANY of it.

◊ Baby wearing may save your sanity. Strap the littlest one to you and go to the park (sit down when you get there).

◊ Don't be surprised when your oldest child's excitement about the new baby wears off and turns into hatred. In their defense, this baby totally killed their only-child vibe and stole their mother. The jealousy is warranted.

◊ Once the littlest one can actually walk, play, and interact, the dynamic in the household will change completely. Usually, it's a good change - enjoy it when it comes!

◊ Prepare yourself to never have any time to make food anymore. Find good (healthy) take-out in your area, ASAP. You'll need it.

◊ Get over yourself and accept help from anyone and everyone who is willing to offer it. If you can unload even one of the kids at any given time - do it. Alternate kids each time so nobody feels neglected. Having one kid to take care of for a day rather than two feels like a goddamn vacation. TAKE THE VACATION!

Story-time with Nikita

LIFE WITH TWO (THE EARLY DAYS)

First babies are scary as shit. You have no idea what you're doing. Everyone keeps throwing the word "phase" out there, but you really can't wrap your head around the concept until the "phase" is over. While you're in the throes of a "phase," it feels like it's never going to end.

The luxury of a second child is perspective. It starts from the day the second line shows up on the pee stick. You know that pregnancy won't be all rainbows and sunshine. You know that you'll have to go to 800 doctor's appointments before you get to meet your sweet babe. You'll show up to ultrasounds mentally prepared for the internal portion of the scan (a big WTF moment with your first). The aches and pains won't be worrisome. The impending delivery won't be (as) terrifying. The initial cluster-feeding won't feel (as much) like cruel and unusual punishment.

You'll smile and nod at all the unsolicited advice you receive, and you'll be able to respond to it with "Yeah, I know. This isn't my first baby." (A retort that shuts up the old guard pretty fast, in my experience.)

Still, even with all of this perspective and experience, trying to simultaneously keep two kids alive and happy (especially if you are expected to do so alone for the majority of the day) can be an absolute shit show at the best of times. It's the juggling act to end all juggling acts: sort one out, the other cries. Calm the crying one down, the other one needs something. Put one to sleep, the other wakes up. Over and over again until it's 3:00 p.m. and you legitimately stop to ponder whether or not you've brushed your teeth today.

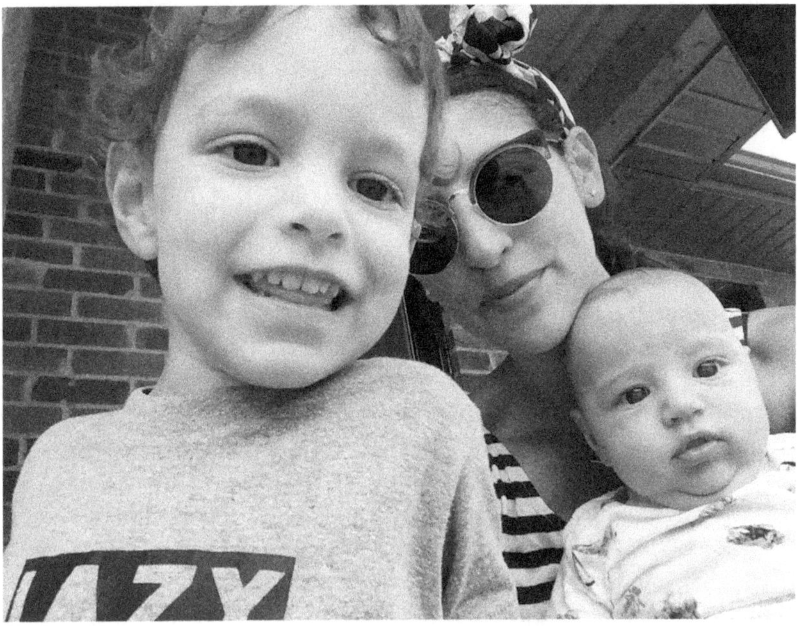

Having two young children is *intense*, and at some point or another, it will likely have you questioning every life decision you've ever made that led you to this moment. HOWEVER (and that's a BIG however), there are also some massive perks that come along with baby number two that cannot and should not be overlooked.

Since this isn't your first rodeo, you're likely to already be a breastfeeding ninja. No longer are you stuffing nursing pillows all around you. You're not stressing about whether or not to wake your baby because he's been sleeping for three hours and you're scared that if you don't wake him, he'll starve. You just shove your boob in his mouth and go about your day.

Since so much of your time is legitimately consumed with making sure the toddler doesn't start swinging from the curtains, you actually don't feel an ounce of guilt for letting the little one chill on his own for a few minutes. When you finally do get back to

Mr. Independent, you'll find him happily playing away, because second children just have a way of figuring their shit out. After all, necessity is the mother of invention.

Oh, and sleep training? Pfft! Here's how that goes with baby number two: put the baby down. Start getting the toddler ready for bed. Baby starts crying. Toddler is already in the bath. Consider leaving the toddler alone in a tub full of water. Nope, not an option. Finish bathing, drying, and dressing toddler. Oh look! Baby has stopped crying and is now asleep. BAM! Sleep Trained.

And OH MY GOD, THE LOVE. No hint of sweetness will go unnoticed with your second. Try for a moment to recall the feelings you had in those first few days with your first child. Remember just staring at his little face? Being totally overwhelmed with emotion and wonder at what you made? That same feeling comes right back with baby number two, minus the shadow of worry and self-doubt that accompanied it the first time around. Imagine all the things you've looked back on and thought, *I wish I had taken the time to really remember this,* or *I wish I had stopped for a minute to truly enjoy that.* Now imagine that you actually got the chance to do exactly that.

My eldest son is responsible for a lot. He taught me how to be a good mama. He taught me to have patience, to prioritize, to be intuitive, and to pick my battles. My second child showed me how damn good the first one made me, and for that, I will always be grateful.

Am I saying it's easy? No. But is it worth it? Abso-fucking-lutely.

HOW TO PRETEND TO BE A FUNCTIONING ADULT WHEN COMPANY DROPS IN

Having more than one kid, especially in the very early days, is messy AF. Nothing sends chills down a mom's spine quite like the announcement that aunt so-and-so wants to come and meet the new baby. And "she'll be there in about twenty minutes."

Shit!

You look around and the house is in complete disarray. It's like when were in college and your parents used to "pop-in" to say hi. They'd always call when they were only a few minutes away (just to make sure everyone was fully clothed). You'd spend the next ten minutes scrambling to ditch old pizza boxes while taking off last night's makeup and trying desperately to get the cigarette smell out of the couch.

Now, instead of pizza boxes, there are balled-up dirty diapers. In place of last night's makeup, there's yesterday's spit-up stain. Instead of spritzing down the smoky couch, you're desperately trying to find a place to stash thirteen unsterilized bottles and enough Legos to build a small village.

The truth is, no matter how many babies we've popped out, we still only kinda have our shit together.

Here's how to make it look like you're a functioning adult when you're faced with a dreaded drop-in:

- **Hide all the toys:** Scrape everything off the floor and shove it all in whatever box it fits in. Neutral-coloured fabric storage containers work wonders for this.

- **Dust corners:** Focus on giant piles of dirt rather than worrying about little specs of dust. Grab the duster or a rag and slide it around the perimeter of the room - that's where the really offensive shit accumulates. If you don't have time to haul the vacuum out, this short-cut will usually do the trick.

- **Give the bathroom sink a quick wipe-down:** When you're done wiping that, use the same cloth to quickly scoop up any tufts of hair that are blowing around on the floor and around the toilet base. Bam! You now reside at the Four Seasons.

- **Close all room doors except for the nursery:** Tidy the nursery by placing all visible clothing into the hamper, stuffies into the crib, and anything else into the closet or dresser drawers. Luckily, the baby's room is the only room in your house people will ever request to see. Show it to them, then politely encourage them to go back downstairs.

- **Get everything off the kitchen counters:** Pick up all the cups and dishes strewn about and put them in the sink (slightly less visible), then spray the counter tops with something that smells nice and wipe that shit down till it shines.

BONUS TIPS:

- If you've got some extra time before your guests arrive, grab a baby wipe and start surface cleaning! Dining-room table, toddler's dirty face and hands, side tables, entertainment unit, dried milk on the wood floors, the stain on your pants, and even your own armpits - baby wipes are surprisingly versatile.

- When your guest arrives, pass off the baby and retreat to the kitchen to put on a pot of coffee and throw some (possibly stale) cookies on a plate. Put the toddler in a high chair and give him one of the cookies to keep him quiet. Enjoy your coffee once it's brewed, and if the cookies are, in fact, stale, just dip them in your cup of Joe like cheap biscotti. Bask in your newfound domestic goddess status.

EXTRA BONUS TIP:

- Always have a spray bottle of water and vinegar locked and loaded. You can literally use it to clean EVERYTHING (floors, glass, countertops, stainless steel, high chairs, upholstery, E.V.E.R.Y.T.H.I.N.G.). It's cheap, it's easy to make, and it's non-toxic (because you know your toddler licks the floors when you're not looking - maybe even when you are looking).

Story-time with Aleksandra

ONE AND DONE

My husband and I were never the couple that was planning for a big family in a newly developed neighbourhood with a two-car garage. We got together while we were throwing parties (our jobs at the time). Our calendars were filled to the brim with blurry nights out, last-minute trips, and all kinds of interesting happenings with interesting people. Naturally, we weren't eager to throw in the towel. Even the idea of having a baby at all was only something we considered after a lot of conversations that basically boiled down to "Let's try. If it works out, we have a kid. If it doesn't, we tried." No pressure.

I got knocked up on our first try.

Fourty-one (and a half) weeks later, we welcomed our baby boy, and it's been a whirlwind of ups and downs since then. Although motherhood didn't start out as an easy adjustment for me, with time I became comfortable in my new mama skin, and found my own way to raise this little man of mine. Things were good. We felt complete.

Except for the occasions when people (friends, family, strangers) dropped their opinions at our feet like a FedEx delivery box.

Thump.

"You can't just have one!"

"HE'S GOING TO BE WEIRD.
ONLY CHILDREN ARE WEIRD."

"Who is he going to play with?
Who will he have when you're gone?"

"That's selfish. You're only thinking of yourself!"

What I wanted to say was:

"Who the hell are you to tell me how to live my life?"

Moms already feel guilty for literally everything, so it's a little odd when people purposefully add to our pile of ever-growing anxiety, even when they mean well. Hearing about what I should and shouldn't do made me feel shitty, and in most cases resentful, too.

For now, *for us*, three is the magic number. We feel comfortable and happy and we can manage with our sanity intact. We are also lucky enough to have some amazing friends who are as close as family, and our kids are already growing up together.

If you're in a similar boat, my advice to you is this: Stick to your guns, and don't let people get you down. It'll be frustrating as hell to have to repeat and defend yourself over and over, but try to focus on more important things, like your family. In the end, you don't want to make any life choices simply to please other people.

Here are a few fun reasons not to have another child. Feel free to throw these back into the face of the baby bullies with a nonchalant smirk and a sprinkle of attitude.

- You won't have to waddle through another pregnancy
- You won't have to give birth, recover, breastfeed, sleep train, or potty train again.
- You won't have to forgo an additional three years of sleep.
- One is about $250,000 cheaper than having two.
- You can fit in one row on a plane.
- You won't be forced to book an all-inclusive vacation or family cruise (shudder).
- Your kid will likely become more independent.
- Your kid will actually enjoy alone time!
- You won't have to drive a mom bus around town.
- You'll be able to stay in your downtown row house.
- Your child will get to choose their own "siblings."
- You'll be able to reap the rewards of a more focused family unit.
- You won't spend your days breaking up fights.
- Your time spent negotiating will be cut in half, as will your grocery, clothing, and entertainment bills.
- You'll have more time and energy for sex.
- You'll spend less time driving the kids back and forth from activities.

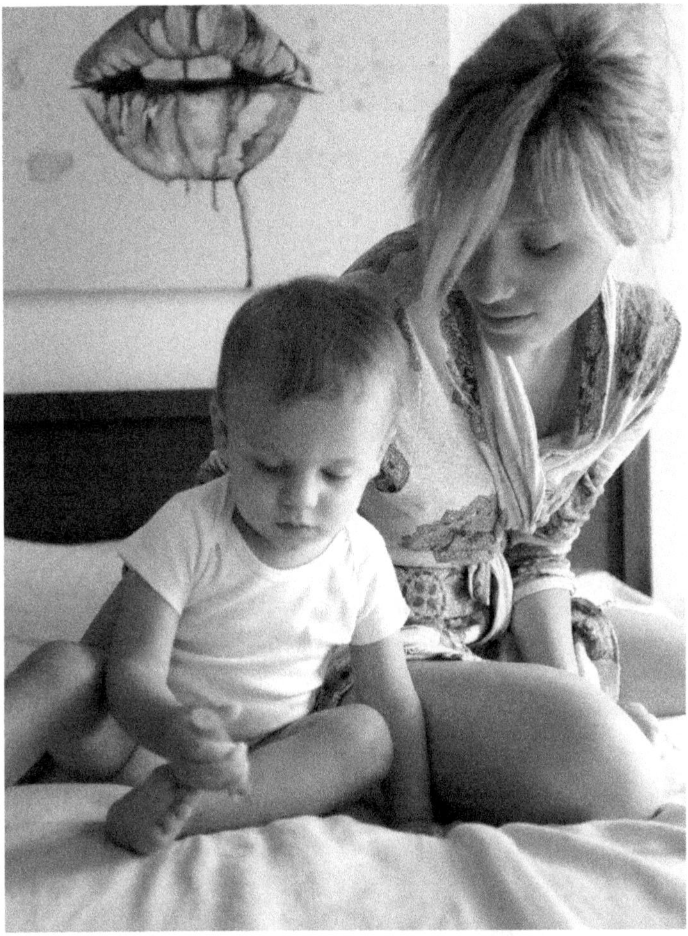

- You'll be more present, since you don't have to split your duties among several children.
- Life will be one-less-human-being calmer.
- Life will be QUIETER, in a good way.
- You'll get to embrace your inner-child and join your kid on the adventure of a lifetime.
- You will get to prove everyone wrong when your babe grows up to be a wonderful, well-adjusted human.

A LETTER TO THE (FURRY) SIBLINGS

Dear fur babies,

Let us begin by saying, We are so sorry.

We know you remember life B.C. (before children): the glory days, when you were the star of the show. We used to take long walks by the beach together, remember? You were given regular baths. You even ate hot, home-cooked meals. You had it all … and then you had a sibling.

When the new human made their first real appearance in your life, they rolled up to the house like they owned the place. They were always in our arms. Always stealing all the attention from visitors - visitors who (back in the day) came over to squish your cute face.

For months to come, the tiny human did nothing but disrupt your leisurely lifestyle. They took up your space in (y)our bed, got you kicked off the couch, and had you pacing around at all hours of the night, trying to escape the piercing sound of their cries.

Then the tiny human became mobile. That's when you discovered that the first few months were only the pre-show for the main event. Ear and tail pulling became the norm. Your food bowls no longer stayed out all day for you to snack on as you pleased. Your daily exercise consisted of escaping a tiny-handed death grip and trying to figure out which toys you could chew on without getting yelled at.

One day, that dreaded human sibling of yours picked up a ball - your ball. They gave it a squeeze and threw it about eight inches from the spot where you were standing. It was a shitty throw (babies are terrible pitchers), but you fetched it anyway; you brought it back and dropped it at their tiny feet. They squealed and threw it again.

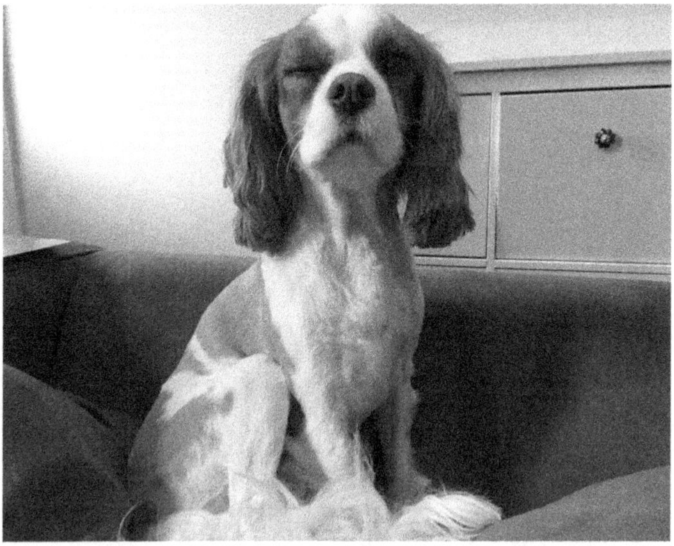

That's when you finally realized that maybe this new sibling of yours wasn't so bad after all. Maybe they would even turn out to be your new best friend.

They will play with you endlessly. They will feed you an entire peanut-butter sandwich from their plate. They will hug you (admittedly tighter than you'd like) and kiss you (admittedly more frequently than you'd like) and adore you like the furry sibling you are to them, every day for the rest of your life.

In return, you'll impart upon them some of that unspoken animal-wisdom of yours: how to be loyal, how to be affectionate, and how to enjoy life. Because of you, they'll understand the value of patience; after all, they will have had to earn your trust. They'll know the difference between gentle and rough, and they'll see what unconditional love looks like.

So, our furry friends, we're sorry to have uprooted your cushy life in the lap of luxury. But we're so grateful that you're here with us during these adventures in early parenthood. We can't imagine doing any of it without you.

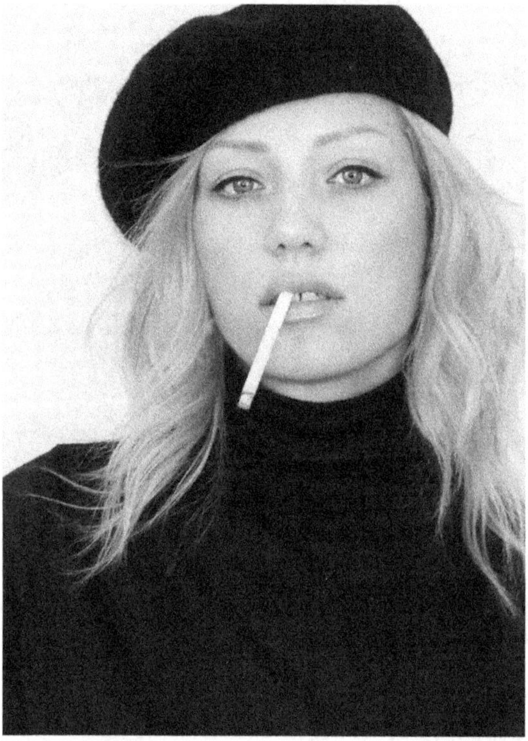

Part 6
ON ESCAPING

"I love my children… I am delighted to see them come and delighted to see them go."

- Mary Wesley

A COMPLETE GUIDE TO TEMPORARY CHILD ABANDONMENT

It's crazy how much energy we mamas use up every day: scanning for potential danger, thinking of stimulating activities, brushing teeth and hair, teaching life lessons, kissing things better, wiping tears, breaking up fights, prepping and administering meals, giving baths, clipping nails, constantly tidying, and doing ten thousand other mom-related mental and physical tasks on a daily basis.

Let's be honest: we all need a fucking break. To get that break, we sometimes need to leave our kids in the capable hands of others, and we should never feel guilty for doing so.

When we leave our kids behind to do something for ourselves, not only are we taking necessary care of ourselves, but the kids reap multiple noteworthy benefits as well:

- They learn that you have a healthy, fulfilling life outside of being their parent (which, in the future, will help them deal with the reality that the world does not, in fact, revolve around them).

- They learn to play by a new set of rules (making them more adaptable to different forms of authority).

- They figure out that a change in scenery is exciting, rather than scary (especially if they spend the night out).

- They get a little time away from you (they're probably just as tired of your shit as you are of theirs).

- They're actually excited to see you once their "vacation" is over!

If you're wondering with whom to dump your kids, grandparents are a good place to start. They *love* feeling like you trust them to keep your kids alive. After all, they kept you alive and you turned out just fine, right? They're free childcare, so now is the time to suck up and shower them with praise for their child-rearing skills. Bonus: Grandparents are often willing to take your kids overnight, which opens up a whole world of free-time possibilities.

The next best option is to find someone you can pay to watch your kids. Mark our words: it will be the best money you've ever spent. Even if it's just to go out for dinner and drinks rather than a whole twenty-four-hour stint, a night out of the house in dry-clean-only clothing will be well worth the hassle. Bonus: you lay down the rules and they stick to 'em (unlike grandparents), because it's their JOB and they want to keep it.

If you can't seem to find a sitter you trust through a friend or family member's recommendation (often the safest and easiest route), try posting in one of your online mommy forums and asking for some highly recommended people in your area. If that doesn't yield any results, go find that nanny you always see at the playground that watches the kid that plays with yours. Many offer part-time / evening help, and she's obviously already good at it.

Failing all that, remind yourself of the dude that knocked you up a while back. He is perfectly capable of being alone with your child for a few hours (and by the way, when he does step up to the plate, it's not babysitting; it's just parenting, and it's his job too).

Have we sold you on a guilt-free night out / weekend away yet?

If you're still on the fence, and the mom guilt is slowly creeping back in because your babe *"really, seriously needs you,"* let us remind you of the benefits you will reap once you successfully escape your household for any amount of time:

- You'll have the opportunity to reintroduce yourself to the woman you were before you took on the title of "mom" (and hopefully feel inspired to bring that fabulous lady back around more often, because in case you forgot, she is AWESOME).

- You'll realize that Tom Ford was wise AF when he famously declared that "time and silence are the most luxurious things today."

- You'll rediscover life's simple pleasures and hone in on forgotten passions. Side note: this may lead to unexpected entrepreneurial ventures! #bossbabe

- By fulfilling your personal needs, you will become a better (and less annoyed / resentful) parent.

- Your relationship with your partner will continue to flourish when you give it the attention (and intimacy) it needs.

- You'll get used to the fact that self-care is worth all the damn time and effort it takes to pull it off – it truly is essential to a happy and fulfilled life.

So please, treat yourself. Check out of your mom-life for short (or long) periods of time. Spend it alone, spend it with your partner, or spend it with your friends. It doesn't really matter, as long as you're spending it without the tiny ball and chain.

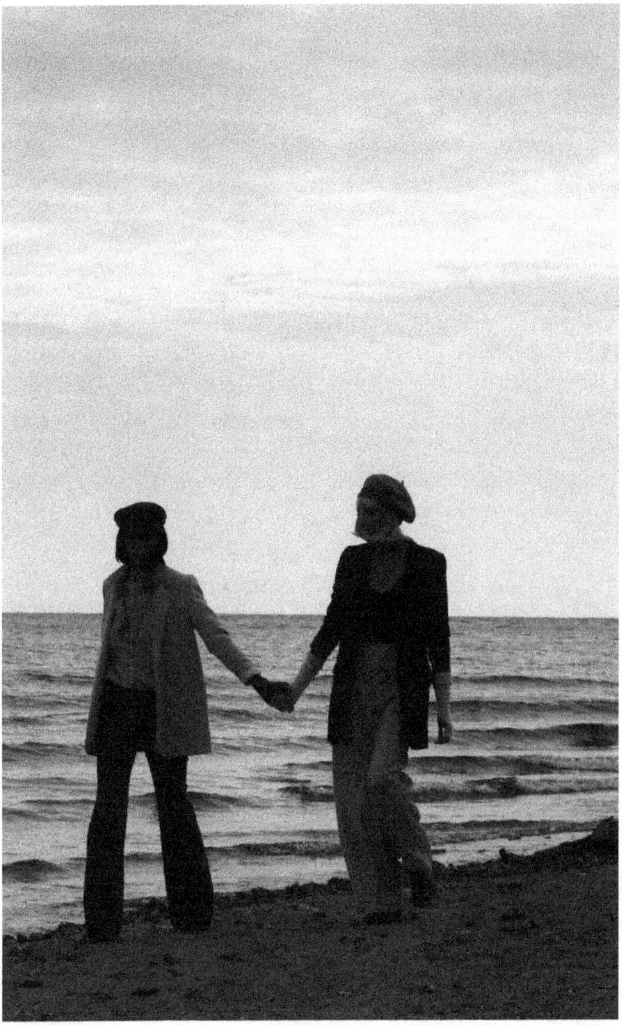

And don't you dare waste even an ounce of energy feeling guilty about it, because upon your return, you will be embraced as a matronly goddess who is once again the centre of her child's universe. Your cooking will be appreciated, your singing regaled, and your mom-skills hailed as some of the best in the land.

Bless.

Story-time with (our friend) Meg Broadbent

MOM'S NIGHT OUT

When my little guy was a few months old, I decided it was high time for a night out. I was on house arrest for almost eight weeks after he was born, and I was getting restless. I wanted to dance. To Beyoncé. On a table. I summoned a few of my girlfriends and we set a date.

The night in question got off to a rocky start when I tried to find something to wear. Getting dressed to go out used to be easy, in that I used to have a body that fit into things. Post-baby, however, was a different story: none of my shirts fit over my enormous milk jugs, and the only jeans that fit me were sweatpants.

After trying on everything in my closet, I finally settled on stretchy black leather leggings and a long black t-shirt. Yes, the t-shirt was baggy, but it had shoulder cut-outs. Flaunt what you still got, right?

The rest of the night went like so:

8:30 p.m.: Glass of wine at home to celebrate the fitting of my body into something other than pyjamas. Go me!

9:00 p.m.: Breastfeed the shit out of baby, so that I can be away from him for as long as possible.

9:25 p.m.: Baby pukes all over the only shirt that still fits me.

9:30 p.m.: Chug two Campari sodas while frantically doing my makeup with one hand and holding baby in the other.

9:45 p.m.: Find another black t-shirt. It may or may not be my husband's. I may or may not care.

10:05 p.m.: Wonder how I'm already so tipsy. Remember that I haven't had more than two drinks in a night since before I got pregnant.

10:10 p.m.: Start dancing to music in my living room. Husband reminds me to leave the house.

10:15 p.m.: Attempt to put heels on. Discover that newly acquired cankles cannot be contained by Alexander Wang's skinny straps. Also, I forget how to walk.

10:30 p.m.: En route to a bar with three of my best girlfriends. I am alive with pleasure and freedom! I am out of the house without my baby! I am buzzed! My hair smells good! Nothing can stop me!

10:31 p.m.: I laugh at something, and to my shock and horror, pee a little bit in my underwear. A chilling vision of things to come.

10:40 p.m.: Tequila shot at the bar.

10:45 p.m.: Sneeze, immediately pee myself for the second time. Ask my doctor friend why this is happening to me. She explains that alcohol aggravates even the mildest case of incontinence caused by a weak pelvic floor, which in turn is caused by pushing an entire football-sized human out of your vagina. WHY, GOD?

11:00 p.m.: Silent tears as I run downstairs to the washroom to investigate. Underwear ruined. No back-up pair. Only solution is to take them off. Never not wearing a diaper in public again.

11:15 p.m.: Decide that the only way to pretend I'm not soaking wet from the waist down is to keep drinking. Buy a bottle of Prosecco. Hear tiny voice inside my head say, "This should end well."

11:30 p.m.: Boobs are rock hard and bigger than my head. I poke gently at one of them and my bra fills with milk.

11:45 p.m.: While walking to our second and final destination (a nightclub a few blocks away), I blow my nose and pee myself for the third time. Remember that I'm not wearing underwear. Discover that leather leggings + pee = hot rubber pants of shame.

12:00 a.m.: Waiting in line. Begin to wonder if everyone can tell that I smell like urine and failure.

12:15 a.m.: Still not inside. I feel like there are giant fluorescent arrows pointing at my head that say "OLD" and "MOM."

12:25 a.m.: My engorged breasts make me look like a blow-up sex doll. Never should have left the house. Zip up coat, ready to throw in the towel and go home.

12:30 a.m.: In defiance of God and nature, we somehow get in. Probably thanks to my blow-up sex-doll boobs. Shot of Jameson to celebrate.

1:00 a.m. – 2:00 a.m.: A blur of dancing and "flirting," aka yelling at strangers "I JUST HAD A BABY AND NOW I'M HERE!" For some reason, do not receive multiple high fives in response.

2:00 a.m.: Corner a group of twenty-something women and tell them never to have children.

2:05 a.m.: Force the bartender to look at pictures of my baby on my phone. "I MADE THIS MOTHERFUCKER WITH MY BODY!"

2:10 a.m.: While aggressively "dancing," fall over onto a couch. Someone asks if I'm okay. I yell, "IT'S MOM'S NIGHT OUT!!!" Again, fewer high fives than expected.

2:30 a.m.: Lights come on. My first thought is that there's a fire drill happening. I warn the DJ. He tells me to go home.

2:45 a.m.: Start walking home. Text literally everyone I know.

3:00 a.m.: Home. Discover that soaking-wet leather leggings are impossible to remove. Manage to get them down to my knees and give up. Waddle to the kitchen like a sad penguin.

3:30 a.m.: Eat everything I can find in the house with my eyes closed. Spill water everywhere on the slow journey from the kitchen to my bedroom.

3:35 a.m.: Turn lights on in bedroom where husband and baby are soundly asleep together. Start taking pictures of them on my phone while loudly whispering how much I love them.

Still got it.

HUNGOVER PARENTING

When you finally make it out of the house for some strange new version of a night of good old-fashioned debauchery, you'll mostly likely have an incredible time. What follows, though, may be the worst twenty-four hours of your adult life.

Because we've made this rookie mistake ourselves, we're giving you some tips on how to survive "the day after" in the hopes that the next time you become over ambitious in the party department, you organize yourself well enough to save your soul from the hell that is Hungover Parenting.

◊◊◊

Your baby will definitely wake earlier than usual, and probably choose that morning to start teething. This is your punishment for trying to have your cake, and eat it too. Do not feel guilty about tossing your usual morning routine out the window and succumbing to the immediate powers of Baby Advil. Pop one back yourself.

Make some strong coffee.

You will feel more nauseous than most hungover ladies, and that's because it's still dark out and you're trying not to puke while mushing up bananas. If you need to vomit, vomit. It won't be the last time your kid sees you do it, and it just makes you more relatable.

During playtime, you will experience severe spins and wonder if your body will actually give up on you before 10 a.m. The playmat is your best friend, and you most certainly need to lay horizontally across it. Give baby an activity, wrap your arms around their waist, and take a three-minute nap.

When you wake up, make more strong coffee.

You will be dehydrated and likely unable to stomach a single thing. This is actually great, because now you only need to prepare food for one human being today. Try to choke down a Mum Mum if you're feeling bold, and chase it with baby's organic apple juice. The sugar will recharge you for the rest of your shift, and it doubles as "hydration."

The hours, minutes, and seconds will pass by as slowly as physically possible. Now is the time to embrace the screen and let the ol' TV be a hero. A few cartoons will not hurt anyone, and this grants you yet another opportunity for a mini nap - except this one can be as long as fifteen to thirty minutes. Amen.

Your baby will choose this day of all days to take a much shorter nap. The one to two hours they've been clocking all week will be a distant memory when a twenty-minute nap brings you face to face with the brutal reality of mom life. Do not attempt to get ANYTHING productive done during nap-time today, as there's no way of knowing how long you have. Every moment counts. Lie down.

Consider making more coffee, but drink water instead. Extra points for sparkling water, which can help your tummy feel less like a trash can.

When your babe is hungry again, don't get ahead of yourself and try to prepare a gourmet feast. Today is a day of basics. Toast, plain yogourt, fruit. The less prep time, and the less scent these foods exude, the better.

Attempt to go outside. Now's not the time to get your cute-mom look on, just muster the cleanest slick-back look you can manage, throw on your biggest and blackest shades, and head out for a lengthy stroll in a low-key area. Bonus: if your baby falls asleep in the stroller, park that bitch (the stroller, of course, not the baby) by a picnic table and tend to your migraine.

While you're out of the house, we should mention that store-bought muffins and croissants are totally considered a suitable meal for you and your whole family today. If you still feel like death, find a hipster cafe and order an Espressino. You're welcome.

You may be tempted to put your baby down for bed earlier today … may the force be with you. This brilliant idea may or may not reap rewards, so attempt at your own risk and expect to deal with an obscene level of volume. We hate to be the bearers of bad news, but the safer bet may just be a little more TV time, darlin'.

If you've somehow managed to make it to the evening hours alive, we urge you to skip your regular bedtime routine as well. Does the baby *realllly* need a bath? Their feet barely touch the ground half the time. Use some wipes and call it a day. Baths require way too much participation on your part right now.

After the child is in bed and you can finally take a proper human shower, really take a moment to acknowledge the consequences of a night out and make some commitments for the next time you unleash the party girl within. Here are our three hottest tips to help you avoid the fresh hell that is hungover parenting in the future:

1. Don't mix drinks. Choose your poison wisely, and stick with it. The cleaner, the better: clear liquor on the rocks with lime is ideal. Sodas, juices, brown liquors, and bubbles all equal a beautiful shade of green in the A.M.

2. Set a hard time cap. Houdini the hell out of whatever event you've chosen to attend when that time comes. Do not, we repeat, DO NOT tell anyone of your plans to exit. When the opportunity presents itself, walk out and don't make eye contact with a single soul. Your text from the cab will read: "I went out for a smoke and felt sick ... sorry babe xx."

3. Plan your nights out strategically. Sleepovers and pre-arranged day-after caretakers are your Get Out of Jail Free Cards in these scenarios. Use them wisely.

Whatever you do, keep those party pants handy, girl. Those tables aren't gonna dance on themselves.

TEN STEPS TO HOME-ALONE HEAVEN

Once you have kids, having the house all to yourself is a rare luxury. Although the scheduling of such a luxury may feel like a deterrent in and of itself, we promise you: carving out the time for some Home-Alone Mama Maintenance is one of those things in life that you will never regret.

Over the years, we've developed a foolproof system that allows us to get the most out of these infrequent occasions, in ten easy steps:

STEP 1:

Pour yourself a cocktail. A real cocktail. One that takes a bit of extra time and energy to stir, shake, and/or garnish." (For ideas, see page 180). Sip in silence.

STEP 2:

Catch up on all the TV shows that your partner HATES. Bask in your uninhibited control of the remote.

STEP 3:

Take a ridiculously long shower. Wash your hair, shave your legs, scrub your feet... Do all the shit you always plan on doing but don't, because normally, as soon as you start to relax, you find yourself leaping out of the shower to attend to (what always turn out to be 'phantom') baby cries.

STEP 4:

Waltz around the entire house naked. Enjoy not having to field questions about why your boobies look sad and whether or not you still have a vagina despite the region being covered in "all that furry stuff."

STEP 5:

Grab the essentials (A.K.A. wine and Nutella). Normally your partner would be all over that wine, and there's no chance your kid would let you crack the Nutella without sharing. Who wants to share their wine or their Nutella? Not you, sister. Not tonight.

STEP 6:

Organize something. You've been left completely unattended and are fuelled with alcohol and sugar. Despite your best efforts at strictly relaxing, you are definitely going to get your tidy on. Whether that's putting the laundry away, lining up the cardboard books in size order, or finally tossing the kids' too-small socks that have been lingering in the sock drawer, a project WILL be completed. Even though it feels lame to admit it, it'll feel freakin' amazing.

STEP 7:

Head outside. Reward yourself for all your hard work by sitting on the back porch with a freshly topped-up glass of something-or-other, or a freshly packed joint. You may decide to treat yourself to some much-needed silence, or listen to the profanity-filled hip-hop that you had to retire from the rotation when your toddler started saying "fuck" in context. Whatever you decide on, savour it.

STEP 8:

Call your girlfriend. The one you never get to talk to, because she's only free after 10:00 p.m. on weeknights. Shoot the shit with her for an hour. Dedicate the first four minutes of the conversation to telling her about the kids, then spend the other fifty-six minutes talking about literally anything else.

STEP 9:

Indulge in some mindless scrolling. Before you hit the sack, park yourself on the couch and grab your phone. Lose yourself in your favourite app for longer than you know you should. Sure, you're on your phone a lot anyway (even when the kids are around; you're no angel), but this way is so much more fun, because it's GUILT-FREE PHONE USAGE. Best night ever.

STEP 10:

Go to bed. Finish off your evening of indulgence by taking your clean, moderately tipsy ass to bed, nice and early. Crawl under the covers, maybe turn on the TV to watch anything but sports highlights, and drift off into uninterrupted dreamland. You've just found Nirvana.

TRAVELLING BY YOUR DAMN SELF

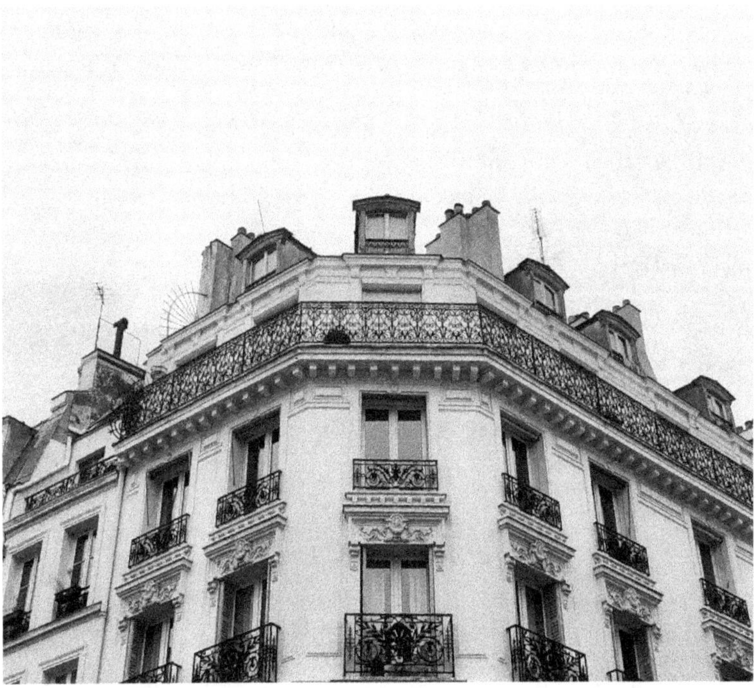

If you are ever able to book a quick trip sans children, do it. Leave them with whoever is willing to be a hero, and go enjoy the luxury of time and silence, guilt free. DO NOT waste precious moments over-thinking and worrying about what's happening at home. As long as your kid(s) are fed and alive, you're good to go.

Bon Voyage!

THE GREAT BACKYARD ESCAPE

There are the obvious escapes, of course, like alcohol, sex, meditation, screaming into a pillow... But we'll let you in on a little secret that you would never expect to come from the likes of us: gardening.

Yes, it's a bizarre and unlikely suggestion, especially considering we have yet to find stylish black gardening gloves, but hear us out.

THE MENTAL PERKS:

Because gardening requires focus, patience, and (our personal fave) silence, it will easily become your new favourite hobby.

As you carefully trim and tidy that random whatchamacallit bush you planted a month back, you'll become very present. You'll ponder relationships (past, present, and future), reflect on your current mental state, and finally have the uninterrupted time and space you need to just THINK. Suddenly, you'll have solutions to those pesky problems that have been keeping you up at night.

THE PHYSICAL PERKS:

If you want to reap the physical benefits of your new favourite pastime, you're going to have to get down and dirty. The more muscle you put in, the better the results will be. Did you know that an hour of gardening can burn anywhere from 120 calories (watering a couple plants) to 450 calories (raking the leaves)? Not to mention you're simultaneously working on a sweet tan.

Gardening has also been linked to lowered stress levels, a stronger heart and immune system, and improved sleep and mental health.

GARDENING 101: GETTING STARTED

If you've never stepped foot in your backyard (other than to sneak an occasional cigarette or pick up dog shit), here's a mini beginner's guide on getting your hands dirty.

You won't need much in terms of tools and machinery, just a basic gardening set that appeals to you on Amazon, a small push mower, and a rake. Wear clothes you give zero fucks about and leave your phone inside.

Begin by cleaning up stray weeds, random dying plants, and anything else that's unappealing. Trim bushes and florals, mow and rake the grass. If you're feeling earnest and want to plant something new, make sure to do some preliminary research on what will most certainly not kill it - be aware of your climate, how much sun you get, or the shitty soil that may need to be replaced. If you're an OCD neat freak who enjoys cleaning, this work will bring you similar gratification.

It is so damn rewarding to sit back in your outdoor chaise and breathe in all that you've accomplished. Before you know it, you will be reaping the benefits of solitude, reflection, beauty, and peace, with a side of dusty pink roses. Practically a private Parisian garden, right?

Get to it, girl. You can thank us later.

*Note: We get that not all ladies are living on acres of rich land. If you're more of a condo-in-the-middle-of-the-city chick, look into community gardening or pretty up that balcony of yours, Euro style.

Part 7
ON MAMA DRAMA

"Patience, n. A minor form of despair, disguised as a virtue."

- Mary Ellen Day

UNSOLICITED
RAPID-FIRE ADVICE

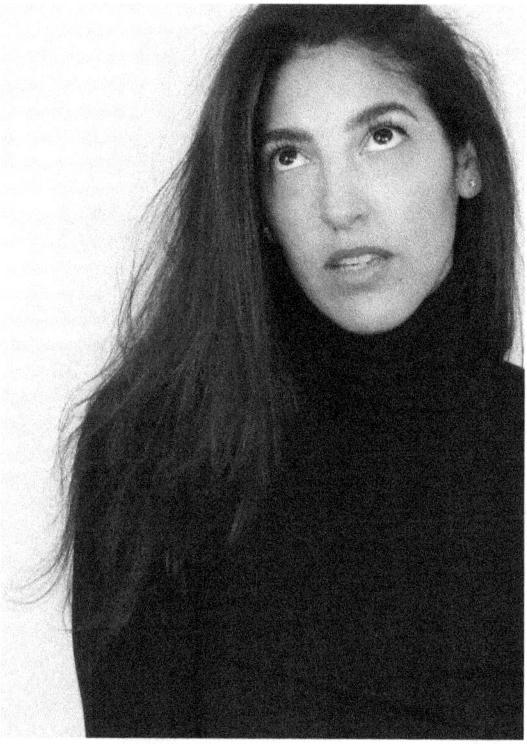

◊ Make open communication with your partner (and all family members, for that matter) your top priority. Having kids is trying, and there is a lot of opportunity for miscommunication, which can lead to fights of epic proportions. Who's got time for that?

◊ Accept that your kids will probably prefer their grandparents to you. They're supposed to. One day, you too will get to be the fun grandparent and feed your grandkids sugar cubes for dessert, but for now, you're stuck with the role of Buzz Killington.

- ◊ Don't fall into the trap of doing *everything* on the domestic front. Just because you're a mom, that doesn't automatically mean you are also a secretary and maid. If you're drowning in chores, remember that the easiest way to get your partner to do more around the house is to stop picking up the slack.

- ◊ Don't bother getting upset with people over petty shit like who was(n't) able to attend a birthday party or a baptism or whatever. It really isn't the end of the world. Sometimes people are just too busy, as you will inevitably be too.

- ◊ Your kids will flip flop back and forth between loving you the most and loving your partner the most. Enjoy the times when you're the chosen one, and don't get all mopey when you're not. This little game is very predictable. It will be your turn again soon, so relax.

- ◊ The concept of "bouncing back" is a load of patriarchal horseshit. You officially have permission to not bounce back, okay? Just bounce yourself into a new normal. As long as you *own it*, it'll be sexy AF.

- ◊ Try not to get super offended when not all public spaces are child friendly, accessible, or even safe. Not everyone prioritizes these little beings, and that's just the world we live in. Don't waste too much of your precious (read: limited) energy being pissed about it.

- ◊ Ignore people's opinions about what you choose to do in your leisure time. Free time is not an easy thing to come by, so when you get it, do whatever the fuck you want. What other people think of you is none of your business. Go live.

EMOTIONAL LABOUR: THE BANE OF OUR MOTHERLY EXISTENCE

Every mother feels the weight of it, yet none of us can seem to figure out how to properly balance the scales.

It's the invisible work that falls on our backs without anyone around us really noticing. It's the mental load: the task of delegating chores, making grocery lists, and figuring out when the plants need to be watered or the dog needs to be fed. It's planning schedules and social calendars, organizing birthday parties and family gatherings. It's remembering every allergy, every milestone, every appointment, every preference, and every fear.

It's a lot to manage, and it's a lot to execute. In the real word, when you're promoted to being a manager or some type of "overseer", *you stop being the labourer.* Why? Because the combination of the mental load (planning) *and* the physical load (executing) is obviously too much to ask of a single person.

Unless, of course, the person in question is a mother.

If you're currently struggling with feeling like all the emotional work you're doing is going unnoticed, please know that we see you, we hear you, and we empathize with you. Luckily, there is an entire army of rebel women (and men!) out there who are fighting for a future in which their daughters and their granddaughters can ditch the mental load (or at least some of it) once and for all.

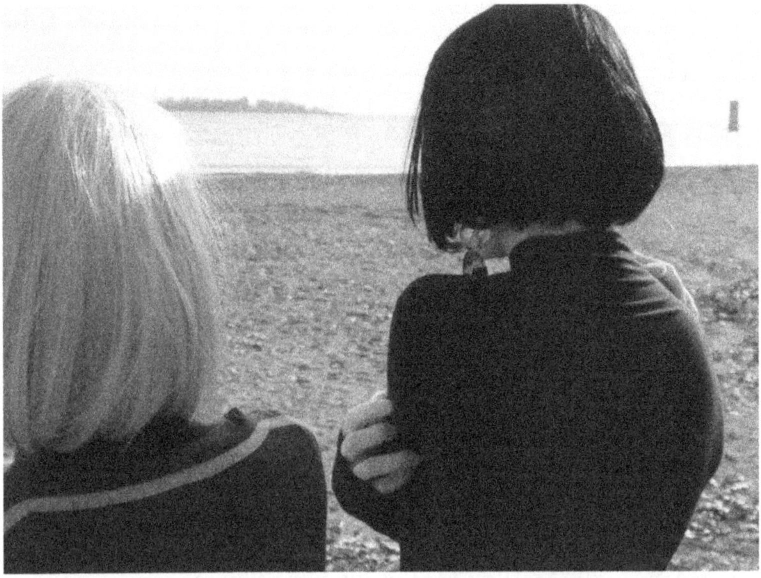

As Rebel Mamas, it is our responsibility to consciously break down gender barriers so that our kids will have the tools they need to balance the emotional-labour scales in *their* future relationships.

We need to expose our kids to a diverse landscape of people (in real life and in books/TV) who are not defined by their sex. They need to understand, through their own experiences, that boys and girls truly are equals, and that categorizing physical work as male and emotional work as female is some arbitrary bullshit.

We need to teach our kids how to take care of themselves and others. Both boys and girls should leave home one day feeling confident in their ability to look after themselves, their living spaces, and (one day) their spawn.

We may not figure out a way to balance the emotional-labour scales in our lifetimes, but we'll be damned if we don't die trying. Our biggest contribution to rectifying this problem may not be something we do, but rather, someone we raise.

BACK TO WORK BULLSHIT

Because you will have been out of the workforce for some time (a year if you're Canadian, and a shitty six weeks if you're one of our neighbours to the south), you may be faced with questions upon your return that will have you pondering what the actual hell is wrong with people.

Here is a list of those questions, accompanied by a few answers you may consider throwing in the mix when you can no longer muster the patience to smile, nod, give a thumbs up, and/or declare, "It's great! Everything's great! I'm enjoying every minute!"

Le sigh.

◊◊◊

"How does it feel to be back in the grind after a year-long vacation?"

Lol. You think that was a vacation? THIS is a vacation. Being at home took WAY more of a mental and emotional toll than any corporate gig ever could.

"Do you just love being a mom?"

If I told you I didn't, would you report me to HR? Fine. I love it. Every moment. Here, check out the scribble my kid made. Talented, right?

"Do you miss them all day? Do you feel bad that someone else is raising them while you're here working?"

I didn't until now! Bless you for bringing it all back to my attention! Is there any wine in this God-forsaken cafeteria?

"Are you still breastfeeding?! How?!!!!"

By pulling out my boobs and pumping in a bathroom stall on every allotted fifteen-minute break, while you suck back a cigarette and take your third trip to Starbucks - that's how.

"Let's skip lunch today and have a quick team brainstorm!"

This is my first meal today, and I will cut you before I let you take it away from me.

"Looks like Bob got the promotion after all; he deserves it, though. He's been really putting in extra hours this month."

How about Bob got that promotion because Bob has a partner dealing with all the at-home bullshit, so he can afford to dedicate some time at the end of the workday without the family home spontaneously combusting? How about handing out promotions to those who really deserve it? *searches frantically in purse for e-cigarette*

"Come on ... just come with us for a few beers after work! You deserve it!"

Sorry lads, bowing out of this one. Not worth my family time, slash, the only forty-five minutes I will get this week to wash AND blow-dry my hair.

"How do you manage it all? A baby, your marriage, your social life ... and now work?"

I don't. I don't manage it at all. I fly through the day by the seat of my pants, hope for the best, and expect the worst. I also drink. *A lot.*

SANTÉ

Prost

γειά μας

乾杯

Cheers

на здоров`я

干杯

Cin Cin

SKÁL

На здравје

KENATS'Y

לחיים

BE NICE TO YOUR MOTHER-IN-LAW (YES, REALLY)

If you have a somewhat rocky relationship with your in-laws, we're guessing it's your mother-in-law who presents the biggest obstacle. We've all been there. Lucky for you, we have some advice on how to deal when your MIL is driving you nuts: let it go.

Let all that rage and annoyance and frustration you're feeling fall away. We promise that if you can master this skill, you will truly be free and so much happier.

The most important thing to do in this situation is to focus on the good. Focus on the common ground between the two of you. You both adore your kid, right? You'd both drop anything for that little guy, do anything to make him happy, yes? Remember that, and try to focus on the love. Whenever you are finding it hard to see the light, do that thing that grown-ass women do and imagine yourself in her shoes.

One day, you will be.

You'll hope that your future son-or-daughter-in-law will appreciate everything you've taught your child about a person's worth.

You'll pray that they will enjoy coming to your house for dinner.

You'll hope that you'll be able to find common ground with them-something you can chat about other than your kid. You'll hope they enjoy your company.

You'll wish they'd trust you more with their children / your grandchildren - just imagine how much love and wisdom you'll have to impart by the time they come along.

You'll hope they don't find you overbearing. You'll do your best to let your child have a life of their own, but how can you possibly guarantee that you won't be wanting to show up, just hoping to be a part of it all?

I mean, come on. Sharing our children? BLEH! Sounds terrible, no? That's what your mother-in-law is doing right now, with you. That's why it's so important that you cut her some slack.

Before she became a grandma, before she became a "MIL", she was a mom, just like you. And as a mom, she had the same dream we all have: the dream of a close, life-long relationship with her child. Facilitating something so profound for another mother is a blessing in and of itself (it's also some hella-good karma).

In the name of full disclosure, we're both some of "the lucky ones" who have great relationships with their mothers-in-laws. We may differ from them in a lot of ways, but we understand them. We empathize with them on a deeper level than we do with most other people. We've taken the time to get to know them, and we appreciate them for who they are. Most importantly, there's mutual respect involved.

Rocky relationships with a MIL are notoriously messy. If you're currently dealing with one, we wish you much strength, because we *know* that shit ain't easy. However, if your bone to pick with your mother-in-law can be categorized in any way as "minor," then please do yourself a favour and let it slide.

Resign yourself to treating her the way you hope to be treated one day. From what we've observed, this mom shit doesn't seem to get any easier with time, so we implore you to lead with a little more empathy when it comes to your mother-in-law. She's doing her best, just like us.

AN ODE TO THE REBEL AUNTIES

When shit gets tough,
When life's not fair,
When baby barf pervades your hair,

When Mama Drama comes on strong,
When Retrograde has done you wrong,
When you just want to drown your sorrows,
And find some hope for bright tomorrows,

When fellow mamas just don't get it,
('cause you're still you - and don't forget it!)
Call your friend who has no spawn,
And rendezvous on your front lawn.

She'll talk you down from off the ledge;
Her faith in you she'll pinky-pledge.

"You're a woman first," she'll tell you straight:
"Martyrdom is not your fate."

For a Rebel Aunty is full of reason
To get you through the icy seasons.
When guilt and doubt hail on your soul,
She'll say, "Some things you can't control."

She'll declare her pride,
And wipe your tears,
And remind you that

you're
not
your
fears.

You'll hug her tight and thank her so.
Could you live without her?
(You don't want to know.)

But rest assured, she's here to stay,
That aunty won't just slip away.

Trust - she knows your value, too;
She wants you there inside her crew,

To show to her the other side,
And give her hope if she decides
To procreate and join your tribe
Of Rebel Mamas far and wide.

But no matter how the tale unfolds,
No matter what the future holds,

In her you'll have a friend for life.
Your ride or die. Your sister-wife.

WHO NEEDS A COCKTAIL?
Go-To Rebel Drinks

A LITTLE IRISH CREAM

Because you are an adult, and it is a legitimate coffee companion.

A CLASSIC ITALIAN NEGRONI

Because it's acceptable at lunch, it opens up your appetite, and doesn't really count as "drinking."

** Stir equal parts gin, Campari, and sweet vermouth with ice. Don't skimp on the orange slice, either.*

SOME FINE RED

Because it's Tuesday night, and that bottle of Barolo isn't going to drink itself.

** Serve slightly chilled in a stemless glass (so you're free to talk with your hands if need be).*

A GLASS OF AMARO NONINO

Because you overdid it at dinner, and this is the only dessert to consider at this point.

** Serve in a chilled crystal glass with an orange peel. Proceed to loosen your shoulders.*

RUM ON THE ROCKS WITH LIME

Because you've finally made it to your beach destination sans baby, and sex is on the breezy horizon.

THE EVER-SO-SLIGHTLY DIRTY MARTINI

Because you need to have a slow and in-depth conversation about life right now.

** Two ounces of (good) Vodka with a splash of (good) olive juice. Quarter-ounce dry vermouth, if it's your vibe. Ingredients are stirred with ice in a cocktail shaker, and strained into a chilled glass. Throw in a few Castelvetrano olives for good luck.*

*** Better yet, get someone else to do it for you at a lovely little restaurant.*

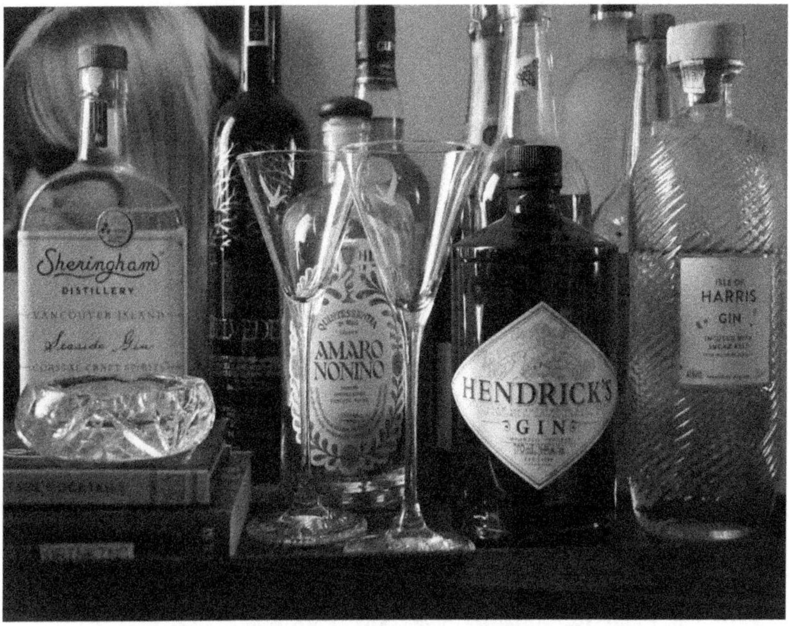

SCOTCH ON THE ROCKS

Because your child has recently learned how to talk back.

** Pairs brilliantly with Dark Chili Chocolate*

AN OG OLD FASHIONED

Because you need to loosen up after an exceptionally shitty week on the job.

** Two ounces (good) Bourbon, a few dashes of orange bitters, a sugar cube, and club soda. Wet the sugar cube using bitters and a splash of soda in a (heavy) glass. Crush it with whatever you can find around the house, add one large ice cube, and pour Bourbon over.*

*** Is also very well enjoyed at the bar of a quaint boutique hotel.*

VODKA ON THE ROCKS WITH LIME

Because you're trying to keep your diet "clean" right now.

TEQUILA SODA WITH LIME

Because you don't need a ruthless hangover, but still want to boogie tonight.

IN CLOSING

A few final remarks before we bid you adieu.

Although it may be hard to fathom this when you haven't washed your hair in days, had a HOT cup of coffee in weeks, or slept in months, early motherhood will be a chapter in your life that you'll look back upon with fondness.

You'll mark the positive changes that it brought about in you. You'll remember it as a time of self-discovery and character growth; as the time when you developed a firm code of morals to live by.

Is it the ethereal skip through the lavender fields you envisioned it to be when you got knocked up? Definitely not. But amidst all the pitfalls and imperfections, there are little bits of pure magic that somehow manage to hold the whole damn thing together.

Feeling the flutter of tiny limbs coming to life inside of your womb: *that's magic.*

Watching a real, live baby emerge through a break in your skin: *that's magic.*

Feeding that baby with milk that flows freely from your breasts: *that's magic.*

Hearing the sound of your baby's sweet voice saying "mama" while touching your face: *that's friggin' magic.*

Being the mother of young children means putting up with a lot of bullshit, but it also means a home that's filled with the sound of tiny feet running through the halls. It means a life filled with endless laughter, where imagination takes priority over reality.

Mama, this is it! These are the times that you will look back on as "the good old days." Although it can be challenging (like, really challenging) to recognize it right now through a haze of boogers, sass, whining, and sleep regressions, these days truly are *good.*

Our hope for you is that you'll embrace all the growth, patience, and maturity that this time has inspired, and use it to be even more of a badass. If you can figure out a way to be both unapologetically yourself and unequivocally a mom, then you're going to be just fine. In fact, you'll be better than fine; you'll be a Rebel Mama.

And so, as the season of Early Motherhood comes to a close, we urge you to stride confidently into the next phase, knowing that no matter what new hurdles come your way, *you've got this.*

FIN.

(... for now)

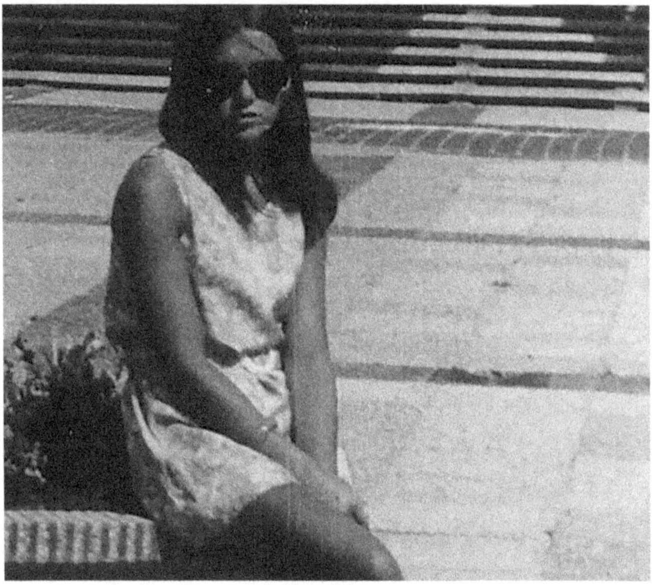

Elizabeth Jassem, circa 1968.

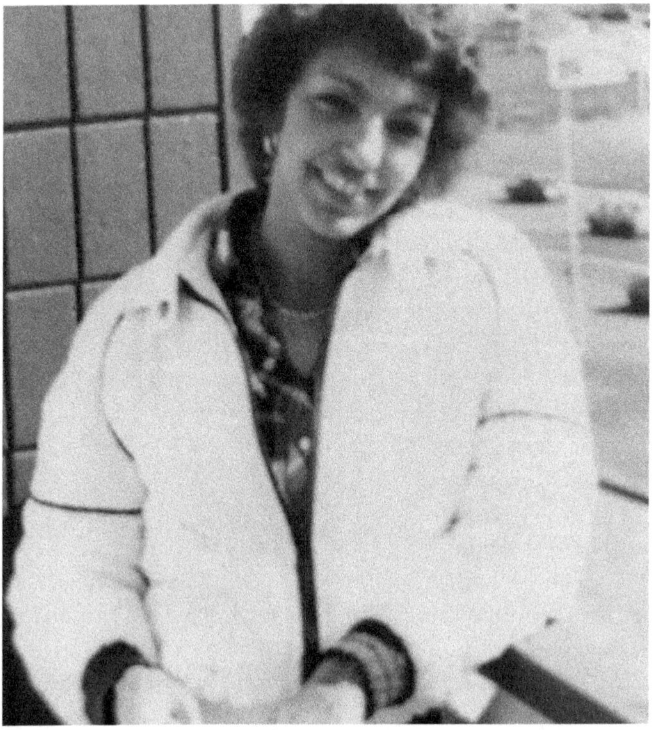

Peta Stanley, circa 1980.

ACKNOWLEDGEMENTS

We would be remiss not to dedicate our first acknowledgement to The OG Rebel Mamas themselves: our moms. Thank you for setting the bar so high for what it means to be a good mother and thank you for holding us to it.

To our kids. You are the driving force of inspiration behind our creativity. Thank you for asking us questions that make us think existentially. Thank you for being hilarious. Thank you for accidentally making us better people. And thank you for showing us how close to death-by-exhaustion a person can get without actually dying - fascinating exercise.

To our partners, Anthony and Jeff. Thank you for so gracefully dealing with the fact that the mothers of your children have chosen to dedicate their time to smashing the patriarchy and conducting business meetings over afternoon Negronis. Also, thank you for being the best papas that Oscar, Beau, and Rocco could ever ask for.

To the amazing Meg Broadbent. Thanks for editing the shit out of this book in the exact filter-free fashion we had hoped for. We will forever cherish your comments in the margins and the cut-throat manner in which you (nearly) cured us of our wordiness. You are a true queen among us.

On the topic of queens, we also want to publicly acknowledge our friend Jen - the first woman to ever introduce to us the concept of absolute, brutal honesty on the topic of motherhood. Jen, your birth story will forever be seared into our brains. Thanks, babe!

To our visual guru, Andrea. Thank you for being one of our most ardent supporters and for blessing us with your creative vision and energy. We're so grateful for you.

To our dear friend, sounding board, and photographer extraordinaire, Ariane. You have been in our corner since the very beginning. Thank you for teaching us how not to look like mega-dorks on camera. That was no easy feat.

To Erica Moore. Thank you for allowing us to share your brilliance with the world. You made this book funny.

To Victor. Real men draw real boobs. Thank you for lending your talents to the cause.

To anyone who contributed to this book by caring for our children, thereby physically allowing us to write it: You guys are the real heroes. Without you, there would be no Handbook for (Cool) Moms. Thank you.

To anyone who contributed to the Kickstarter Campaign that launched this project: You paid for this shit! Thank you for believing in us with your wallet.

To Soho House: Thank you for keeping us hydrated and fed and providing us with dimly lit corners within which to hide and/or host spontaneous lunch parties.

To Google: Thank you for the invention of Google Docs, which are essentially the glue that holds the two of us (and our brains) together.

To our friend Mary J: Thank you for all the great epiphanies.

To our Dads. Did you think we forgot you? We didn't. We could never. Thank you for your unwavering support since the beginning of time.

And finally, to all the Rebel Mamas who came before us and paved the path upon which we walked in creating this platform: We understand what a privilege it is to have this space, and we will never take for granted how hard you fought to break down barriers so that we could write a book of this nature.

The mad woman has officially descended from the attic.

xx
Aleks & Nikita

CREATIVE CONTRIBUTORS

Andrea Xavier. Creative Director. Photographer. Toronto
Featured on pages: xxi, 70, 98, 103, 115, 127, 163, 174-175

Ariane Laezza. Photographer. Toronto
Featured on pages: xv, 2, 7, 24, 54, 100, 106, 132, 143, 146, 151, 168, 171

Briony Douglas. Photographer. Toronto
Featured on pages: 38-39, 84-85, 190

Erica Moore. Writer. Toronto
Featured on page: 40-43

Meg Broadbent. Writer. Editor. Toronto
Featured on page: xi-xiii, 152-155

Victor Xavier. Illustrator. Toronto
Featured on page: 32-33, 119

Oh yeah, and us. We threw a couple of photos in here too.
Featured on page, 57, 181, 184 (Aleks) and 135, 145, 185 (Nikita).

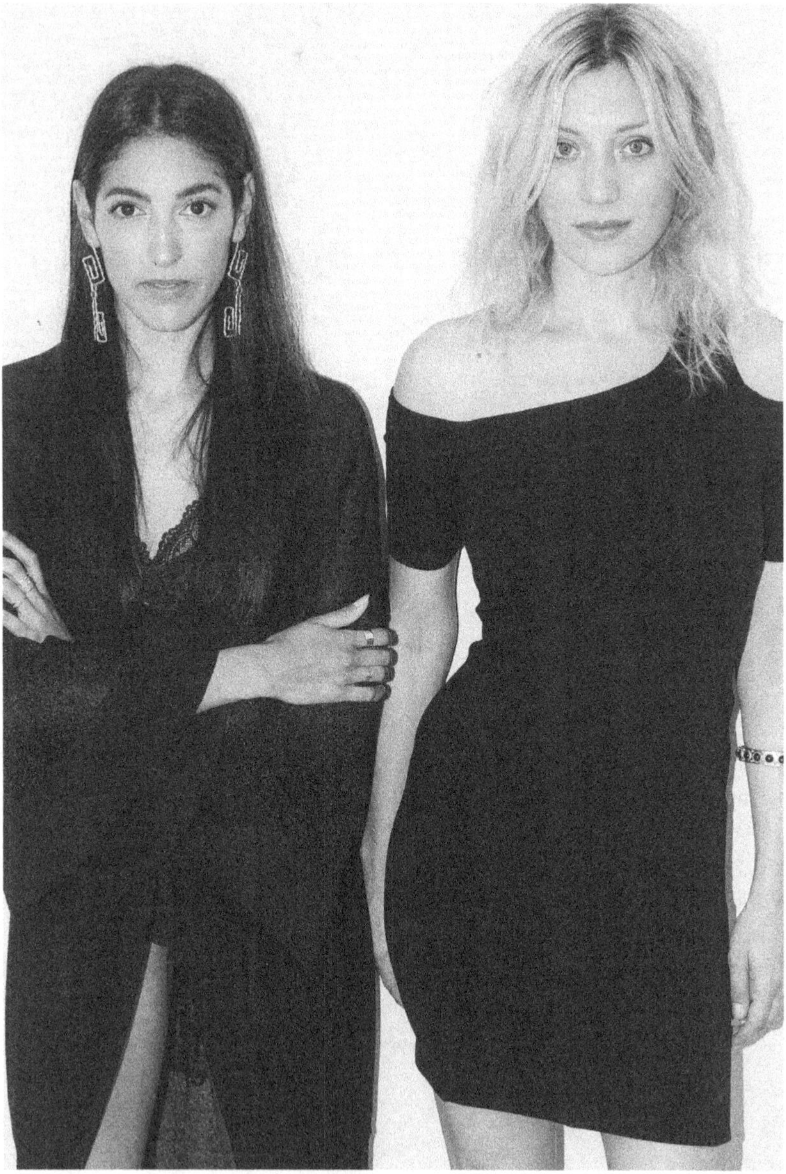

ABOUT THE AUTHORS

Aleksandra Jassem (the blonde) and Nikita Stanley (the brunette) are a pair of former party-girls who got unintentionally pregnant within weeks of each other and went from acquaintances to best friends in a (fetal) heartbeat.

In 2014, the two unlikely moms combined their talents and mutual disdain for the typical mommy-blog B.S. and created The Rebel Mama(.com). Adored by cool moms the world over, the smart and edgy online publication creates a safe and judgement-free space that's known for sharp wit and brutal honesty.

Between the two of them, Aleks and Nikita are mamas to three kids, a dog, and a cat. They reside in Toronto, Canada and survive (almost) exclusively on peanut butter sandwiches, Napolitano pizza, and coffee. So much coffee.

CPSIA information can be obtained
at www.ICGtesting.com
Printed in the USA
LVHW081952310319
612487LV00001B/1/P

9 781525 524950